ADRENALINE JUNKIES & SEROTONIN SEEKERS

ADRENALINE JUNKIES & SEROTONIN SEEKERS

Balance Your Brain Chemistry to Maximize Energy, Stamina, Mental Sharpness and Emotional Well-Being

MATT CHURCH

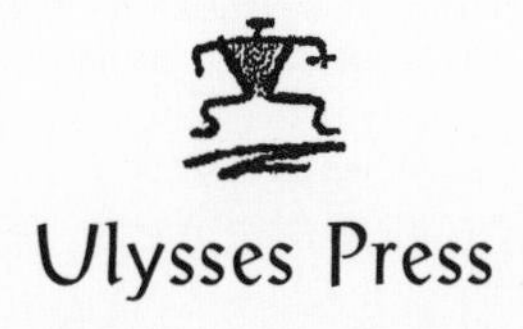

Ulysses Press

Published by Ulysses Press
P.O. Box 3440
Berkeley, CA 94703
www.ulyssespress.com

First published as *The High Life* in Australia in 2002 by ABC Books

ISBN 1-56975-437-3
Library of Congress Control Number 2004108851

Printed and bound in Canada by Transcontinental Printing
10 9 8 7 6 5 4 3 2 1

Interior designed by i2i design
Cover designed by Jake Flaherty

Distributed in the United States by Publishers Group West
and in Canada by Raincoast Books

Please Note
This book has been written and published strictly for informational purposes, and in no way should be used as a substitute for consultation with your medical doctor or a health care professional. All facts in this book came from medical files, clinical journals, scientific publications, personal interviews, published trade books, self-published materials by experts, magazine articles, and the personal-practice experiences of the authorities quoted or sources cited. You should not consider educational material herein to be the practice of medicine or to replace consultation with a physician or other medical practitioner. The author and publisher are providing you with information in this work so that you can have the knowledge and can choose, at your own risk, to act on that knowledge. The author and publisher also urge all readers to be aware of their health status and to consult health care professionals before beginning any health program.

Lex, I am higher because of all you do.

contents

Better living through chemistry.

DU PONT CORPORATE SLOGAN, 1960S

1

balance your body chemistry

two natural highs — one quick one slow

You can get a natural high in two ways — one from adrenaline, which makes you feel switched on for short bursts; the other from serotonin, which makes you feel calm and comfortable for longer periods. The real natural high comes from an appropriate balance of both adrenaline and serotonin — you need to conserve adrenaline to have access to the "rush" under pressure, as well as develop a lifestyle that boosts serotonin levels to experience the comfortable, calm, relaxed, "blissed out" state it creates.

the big 5 natural chemicals

Each chemical in your body serves many functions, all helping in their own way to achieve a natural high. **Adrenaline** gives the speed and confidence you need during busy times. **Serotonin** serves to make you comfortable, relaxed and happy. **Cortisol** is a back-up for when you run out of adrenaline and it is useful in times of enormous stress. Without **melatonin** you are unable to sleep deeply and restore your own natural chemical balance. **Insulin** is the key to controlling your sugar levels — too much or too little insulin leaves you either manic or knocked out.

Your body uses all these chemicals in a delicate balance — as you decrease one you increase the other, much like the balance between the clutch and accelerator when you change gears in a manual car. For example, because adrenaline partners with cortisol, when you're running low on adrenaline, you increase your reliance on cortisol, but dealing with stress by using cortisol leaves you feeling exhausted, uptight, edgy and cranky.

Adrenaline

ı)) *I've always seen myself as a tough negotiator — I find the chase so much more satisfying than the win. In the middle of closing a major deal all my senses are highly tuned, I may have been working late nights for weeks and "dial a pizza" is speed dial #1 on my mobile. I love it! It's addictive and I tend to churn and burn those around me in my manic search for the next fix. I know I'm addicted to the high but it seems pretty harmless.*

The natural chemical of speed, adrenaline gives you a "rush." When you're on adrenaline you think quickly, eat quickly, talk quickly and finish other people's sentences for them. Your pulse quickens and you become polyphasic, able to concentrate on more than one thing at a time. It's a high-performance confidence chemical that helps you avoid pain, stay focused and handle many tasks at once.

Eating red meat and fatty foods, drinking coffee, mentally pumping yourself up and handling crises all give you the "rush" of an adrenaline high.

Serotonin

ı)) *There are only a few times in my life when I can say I was truly happy. I remember one such time so clearly that I now use it as a benchmark for good living. I was with my partner in Noosa on Australia's*

Sunshine Coast — one of the prettiest places on earth. Jenny had just bought some art that we'd been admiring for days and we were sitting in the sun sipping a great coffee from Aroma's. I was so content and didn't feel the need to be anywhere else. The rest of the holiday flowed in much the same way. I try every week now to rediscover that calm "blissed out" feeling. Sometimes it's playing with the kids, sometimes it's reading the paper — often it comes about from a spontaneous sit on a park bench. To me a successful life will be discovering how many more moments like that holiday I can achieve.

Serotonin is the chemical of happiness. When you feel calm, relaxed and satisfied, there is serotonin in your brain. You need abundant supplies of this chemical for long-term enduring motivation. High levels of serotonin means your appetite is in control and your weight stays constant rather than fluctuating. You feel you can cope with change and you're able to tolerate what might normally irritate you.

Many people have a genetic predisposition for low serotonin, although most experts agree that lifestyle and thought habits probably play a greater part in influencing amounts of serotonin. Getting deep sleep, eating well, exercising regularly and observing how you think will set you up for a serotonin high.

Cortisol

I've been snapping at people lately and can't explain it. I love my husband yet every night I say something that starts an argument. I guess we've been under a lot of pressure lately with the sale of our house and all the weekends running in and out of open houses looking for a new place to live. Add the challenges of a newborn and the lost sleep, it's no wonder I'm stressed out! I've stopped swimming laps and am putting on weight. I think one thing and then say something completely different. I'm not even laughing very much anymore.

SNAPSHOT

Adrenaline makes you feel "switched on" in short bursts.

Serotonin makes you feel calm and comfortable for longer periods.

Cortisol stops you feeling calm and leads to anxiety.

Melatonin helps you sleep well at night and wake up with both adrenaline and serotonin.

Insulin is responsible for the ups and downs, the sugar highs and lows.

If adrenaline is a high-octane daily renewing fuel, cortisol is the always-present alternative. When someone talks about being stressed, they usually show the symptoms of someone who has too much cortisol in their system. With too much cortisol you get irritated, uptight and edgy, and find yourself angry most of the time. Constant stress, high crisis or even just an anxious temperament can all lead to an abuse of your cortisol emergency system.

Melatonin

A great night at a friend's place recently ended up going on later than I would have liked — I love to get to bed by about 10.30 each night. Victor had just bought an espresso maker and insisted we all try a little of each flavor bean. I couldn't sleep that night. It took me until 4:00 a.m. to be able to even close my eyes. I then spent the whole of the next day walking around as if I had jet lag. That was over a week ago and I still don't think I've fully recovered.

Melatonin works hand in hand with serotonin. Serotonin makes you happy during the day while melatonin makes you mellow and sleep deeply during the night. With good supplies of melatonin you'll wake up restored.

Insulin

Ever since I can remember I've known not to drink too much Coke. One day as a kid I drank a bottle in one sitting and could not sit still. I felt so sick I haven't wanted to touch any since. At a course I went to I learned about insulin for the first time and know for sure I'm sugar sensitive. Every day I'd been having boiled rice for lunch and wondering why I felt so tired in the afternoons — now I know.

To prevent brain sugar going out of control the body produces insulin. Lifestyle factors, or possibly a genetic predisposition, make some people more sugar sensitive than others. For many, a simple awareness of their sugar sensitivity can change energy levels dramatically.

Brain versus body chemistry

The serotonin high and adrenaline high are brought about by two distinct chemical processes — brain chemistry and body chemistry. Brain chemistry is subtle and often slow to respond, while body chemistry is more direct. A serotonin high uses brain chemistry while an adrenaline high uses body chemistry.

Brain chemistry basics

Brain chemistry works via the various neural pathways that direct behavior.

The human brain is made up of a network of 100 billion *neurons*, special cells that communicate with one another via the *neurotransmitters*.

Researchers have identified hundreds of neurotransmitters that regulate nerve functions, including memory, appetite, mental function, mood, movement and the wake–sleep cycle. Among these neurotransmitters are serotonin, dopamine, norepinephrine, endorphins, acetylcholine and GABA. What you eat and when you eat it, along with exercise and other behavior, can all affect neurotransmitter production. The neurotransmitter serotonin, a star player in achieving a naturally high life, links up neurons making you feel happier and less depressed.

What do you need?

- Are you getting enough sleep?
- Do you eat well?
- Are you active and exercising regularly?
- Do you enjoy the way you think and are you happy with your behaviors?
- Are you dealing with the stresses in your life?
- If you answered "no" to any of these you can balance your body chemistry and achieve a higher life through simple strategies.

Brain cells are separated by gaps, or synapses, which act as firebreaks against overstimulation. These gaps allow the brain to control whether a message will be sent or not. At the gap between two brain cells, several different neurotransmitters sit in storage sacs waiting to be released. It is the neurotransmitter that closes the gap between two cells.

Once a neurotransmitter has traveled the gap between brain cells it needs to find a matching receptor site. If it secures a spot on the other side, the brain's messages will get through. If it doesn't there's a system breakdown, which manifests itself in a multitude of ways including depression, anxiety or even food cravings.

Body chemistry basics

While neurotransmitters affect brain chemistry, hormones affect body chemistry and behavior and are less contained than brain chemistry.

Hormones are generally produced in the endocrine glands (which are found in different parts of the body) — the pituitary gland, the thyroid gland, the pancreas, the adrenal cortex and medulla, and the ovaries or testes.

Body chemistry has a direct, and often immediate, impact on performance. At the adrenal cortex, the hormones adrenaline and cortisol are released, speeding up the heart rate and the flow of blood and oxygen to working muscles. This makes the fight or flight response possible and makes you all but immune to pain. But an overuse of this emergency system will make you uptight and exhausted, rather than alert and focused. Constant abuse of your fight or flight mechanism blunts the chemical response. Your body begins to accept the pressure as normal and continues to supply the "rush" at a diminishing rate.

Many chemicals, such as adrenaline, norepinephrine and melatonin, work across both systems. They can act both as neurotransmitters in the brain and hormones in the body.

how neurotransmitters work

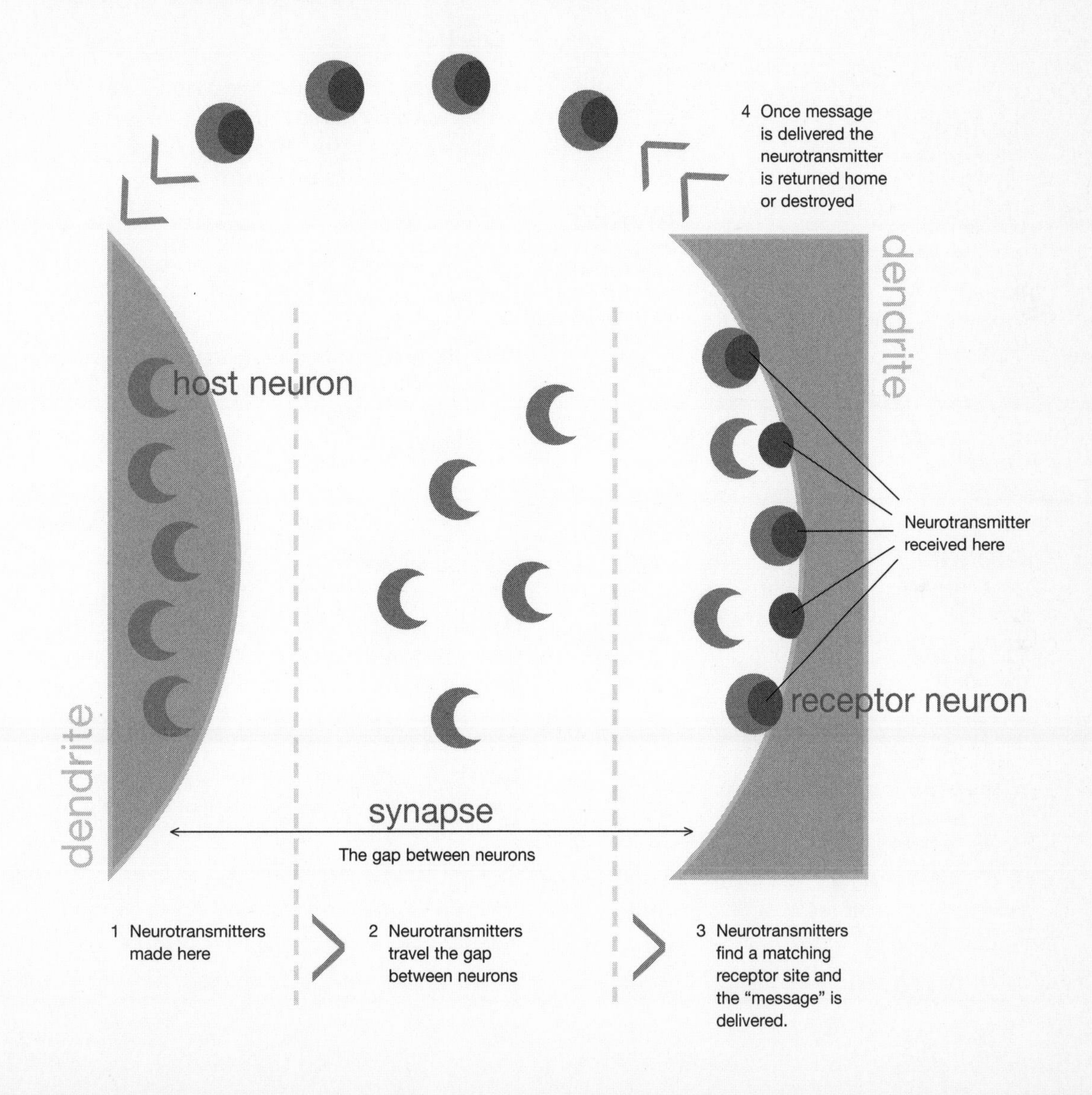

endocrine system

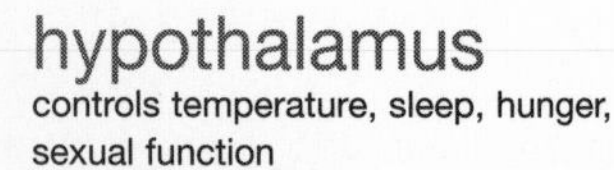

hypothalamus
controls temperature, sleep, hunger, sexual function

pituitary
controls release of hormones

pineal
important in the production of melatonin

thyroid
growth and development of body tissues and calcium levels in the blood

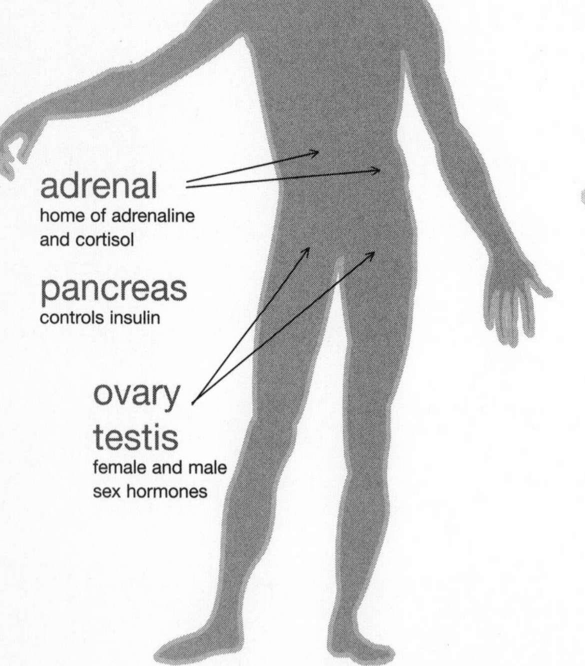

the 5 key lifestyle factors

How well you sleep, the food you eat, how active you are, the way you think and how you manage stress are the key areas of your life affecting internal chemistry and your chances for a high life.

‹1› How well you sleep

When you sleep your body restores chemical balance, repairs muscle tissue damage, processes memories from the day and stores into long-term memory those things you perceive as important.

‹2› The food you eat

Generally, a bad basic diet will create a state of stress for your body, which is forced to use emergency system chemicals to suppress appetite and give you the power you need to get through the day. The food you eat also has a direct and often immediate effect on your internal chemistry — certain foods will elevate your serotonin levels while others may cause an adrenaline spike.

How active you are

Like food, exercise has both a foundation and a trigger effect. A good fitness foundation allows you to manage pressure with less adrenaline response and certain exercises can increase your serotonin production. You can also use exercise to burn off excess stress chemicals and rapidly restore your internal balance.

The way you think

Body chemistry is influenced by how you think. If you're scared, adrenaline kicks in, when you're sad, serotonin levels are decreased. Controlling how you think is an essential step in the balance of body chemistry and the pursuit of a naturally high life.

The way you manage stress

Even though stress throws your chemistry out of balance, you can improve your ability to tolerate higher stress. Managing your stress is an essential step to ensuring chemical balance.

your current chemical balance profile

At any given moment you're using a mix of all the five big chemicals in your body — adrenaline, serotonin, cortisol, melatonin and insulin. If you're under stress, unhappy or just coping with everyday life, you lean on some more than others. Using your five key chemicals in a balanced way means you'll stay naturally high more often and for longer periods.

The following questions associated with each of these five chemicals are a useful guide as to whether you rely on a particular chemical or set of chemicals.

As you go through the questions, particularly take notice of those you answer with a "yes" as this indicates an over reliance on one or two of the chemicals. Too much reliance on one or two chemicals is an early warning of high stress. A high number of "yes" scores in all five means you're a candidate for burnout.

Profile yourself every few months, using the answer sheet on the following pages. Your chemicals of choice may change over time depending on what is happening in your life at the time you do the profile.

Adrenaline

1 Do you find yourself eating more quickly than others around you? ❍ yes ❍ no
2 Would you eat lunch at your desk more than 3 times a week? ❍ yes ❍ no
3 Do you often drive fast even if you're not in a hurry? ❍ yes ❍ no
4 If you had 3 weeks to finish something would you still leave it until the last minute? ❍ yes ❍ no
5 Is it hard to imagine yourself doing nothing? Just sitting — no TV, no reading, absolutely nothing — for an hour a day? ❍ yes ❍ no

YOUR SCORE ❑ yes ❑ no

If you answered "yes" to more than 3 of these questions you're probably an adrenaline junkie.

Serotonin

1 Do you find that a cloudy day affects your disposition? ❍ yes ❍ no
2 Do you eat after you've had an argument? ❍ yes ❍ no
3 Do you crave sugar mid-afternoon? ❍ yes ❍ no
4 Do you snack mainly on carbohydrates rather than proteins? ❍ yes ❍ no
5 When stressed, are you likely to have mood swings? ❍ yes ❍ no

YOUR SCORE ❑ yes ❑ no

If you answered "yes" to more than 3 of these questions you're probably a serotonin seeker.

Cortisol

1 Can you imagine driving home thinking loving thoughts about your kids only to yell at one of them when you walk through the door? ❍ yes ❍ no
2 Do you think you snap at people more than you should? ❍ yes ❍ no
3 If you're a regular exerciser and miss a workout for a couple of days, do you feel a creeping edginess? ❍ yes ❍ no
4 Do you often find yourself twitching and foot tapping in meetings where you're required to listen rather than speak? ❍ yes ❍ no

5 When stressed, do you become angry, sad, afraid or guilty more often than you think you should? ❍ yes ❍ no

YOUR SCORE ❑ yes ❑ no

If you answered "yes" to more than 3 of these questions you're probably getting cranky on cortisol.

Melatonin

1 If you drink coffee in the evening do you feel it affects the quality of your sleep? ❍ yes ❍ no
2 When you spend a day in the sun do you sleep better at night? ❍ yes ❍ no
3 If you're stressed during your day, do you find it hard to sleep well at night? ❍ yes ❍ no
4 Do you think you suffer from jet lag more than other people you travel with? ❍ yes ❍ no
5 Would you love to travel with your own bed and pillow whenever you were away from home? ❍ yes ❍ no

YOUR SCORE ❑ yes ❑ no

If you answered "yes" to more than 3 of these questions you probably need to increase melatonin levels.

Insulin and sugar sensitivity

1 Do you find you're sleepy after lunch more often than not? ❍ yes ❍ no
2 Does a sweet snack give you a noticeable rush or temporary high? ❍ yes ❍ no
3 Is your day a roller coaster of energy and mood — one moment you can focus with great clarity and the next moment you're clueless? ❍ yes ❍ no
4 Are you tired a lot of the time? ❍ yes ❍ no
5 Does your attention wander? Do you have trouble concentrating, particularly when stressed? ❍ yes ❍ no

YOUR SCORE ❑ yes ❑ no

If you answered "yes" to more than 3 of these questions you may have a sugar sensitivity.

Signs of imbalance

The 5 big chemicals are natural and are created by your body. If we rely too heavily on one, we can create a fatigue or imbalance in our internal ecology. This is fairly easy to identify.

Adrenaline imbalance

Adrenaline fatigue leaves you flat, apathetic and feeling lackluster. You feel like you are running on empty. The need for speed is still present, the ability to pick yourself up is not.

Serotonin imbalance

As serotonin is responsible for a calm comfortable feeling, imbalance is often identified as restlessness or a sense of dissatisfaction. An extreme imbalance is indicated by depression or sadness, a propensity for violence or aggressive behavior.

Cortisol imbalance

A little cortisol helps you maintain a level of healthy anxiety, a natural caution when pushing yourself out of your comfort zone. Too much and you become hypersensitive, paranoid and snappy.

Melatonin imbalance

Feeling jet lagged when you have not been anywhere is a good indication of a melatonin imbalance. Finding it hard to get up in the morning and a messed-up sleep-wake cycle are other signs.

Insulin imbalance

Sleepiness after food, easy weight gain and a lack of focus or concentration are all indicators that there may be a problem with your sugar sensitivity and insulin regulation.

balance your body chemistry

By balancing your body chemistry you'll avoid burnout and give yourself maximum opportunity for a naturally high life. Your current chemical balance profile will change over time — you may be under huge stress during the first half of the year and incredibly focused in the second half. By checking your profile regularly you'll get early warning of any imbalances so you can take the steps necessary to bring order back to your profile.

1 You can achieve two kinds of natural high — the adrenaline high or "rush" and the serotonin high or "bliss." An adrenaline high is short lived but useful during times of stress. The serotonin high is more enduring and creates a calm comfortable feeling.

2 The serotonin high is controlled by brain chemistry — neurotransmitters and brain cells working together over time to improve your mood. The adrenaline high is controlled by body chemistry through a process that uses glands, organs and hormones to deal with life events, often overreacting to stress and exhausting itself.

3 There are five big chemicals that affect a natural high. Adrenaline is responsible for speed and confidence, serotonin for calm and happiness, cortisol for anxiety and stress, melatonin for sleep and recovery, and insulin for energy and weight loss.

4 There are five lifestyle factors that influence these chemicals and are the keys to a natural high: how you sleep, what you eat, how active you are, the way you think and behave and how you manage stress.

lights

5 Your current chemical balance profile can help you identify which lifestyle practices you need to modify to balance your body chemistry and achieve a high life.

Not snow, no, nor rain, nor heat,

nor night keeps them from accomplishing

their appointed courses with all speed.

HERODOTUS

2

the big 5

SNAPSHOT

The adrenaline highway

High adrenaline lifestyle › Breathing becomes quicker › Blood thickens and pulse races › Sugar is dumped › Cholesterol goes up › Appetite is suppressed › Adrenaline runs out

The serotonin roundabout

Low serotonin lifestyle › Hunger changes › Cravings for sugar › Stress threshold is lowered › Apathy increases › Thinking becomes distorted › Sleep is disturbed

The cortisol gridlock

High prolonged stress › The cortisol gridlock › High prolonged stress › Reliance on cortisol increases › Inflammation decreases › Muscle tension increases › The fat cells open › Blood sugar increases › Feelings of fear, edginess and anxiety

The melatonin off ramp

Sunlight makes melatonin › Body clock is set › Darkness triggers melatonin › Caffeine may get in the way › Serotonin should switch off › Temperature plays a part › Deep sleep restores body balance

The insulin crash zone

Sugar, a source of fuel › The body selects sugar › Insulin is released › The fat cells open › Brain proteins cross over › Cholesterol goes up › Blood sugar is lowered

the adrenaline expressway

1 High adrenaline lifestyle

Adrenaline exists to give you a rush when you need it. As you go through your day, events or thoughts (stimulating events) trigger the release of adrenaline (unless you're adrenaline depleted already). These thoughts may arise from good and bad stress events. For example, adrenaline is released when you become excited as well as when you're under pressure to get something done.

2 Breathing becomes shallow

In an attempt to get more oxygen into your lungs you breathe more quickly, a kind of hyperventilation. This breathing is shallow and ineffective. But filling your lungs with oxygen is only the first step. To get oxygen from the lungs into the blood stream you need a high aerobic capacity.

3 Blood thickens and pulse races

In response to adrenaline being released your blood thickens — another aspect of the fight or flight mechanism, originating from the early days of evolution to prevent you bleeding to death after fighting a tiger. This explains stress-related blood pressure.

As your heart works to deliver oxygen-rich blood to your working muscles, it beats faster. Your muscles are then able to go to work, lashing out at the tiger or moving those large muscle groups in your legs and arms as you run back to the safety of your cave.

4 Sugar is dumped

Along with oxygen, your muscles need glucose or sugar to help you fight or flee. The liver dumps glucose into your blood supply — your muscles use this in your physical response to stress. But if you sit in your car in traffic rather than running away this sugar hangs around unused.

Your body senses that blood sugar is out of control and releases insulin. Insulin is an aggressive substance — its role in regulating sugar is driven by the need to keep brain glucose levels even. Often your body will dump a great deal of insulin in response to a relatively small amount of sugar. If you have low blood sugar, your body would rather you were asleep; if you have high blood sugar you feel "hyper."

5 Cholesterol goes up

Arteries carry blood away from your heart. Insulin is so aggressive at fighting sugar that your body increases the cholesterol coating inside your arteries and protects other parts of your body from being damaged by the insulin. This explains high cholesterol in response to high stress and why eating highly refined sugar is not recommended if you're trying to lower cholesterol.

6 Appetite is suppressed

Adrenaline suppresses your appetite temporarily. If you skip breakfast in response to the stimulation of getting on with the day, your hunger is deferred.

7 Adrenaline runs out

While the exact amount of adrenaline in the body varies from person to person, there is a finite amount available each 24 hours. Although your body doesn't completely run out of adrenaline, the effects of depleted adrenaline are the same as not having any at all.

the adrenaline expressway

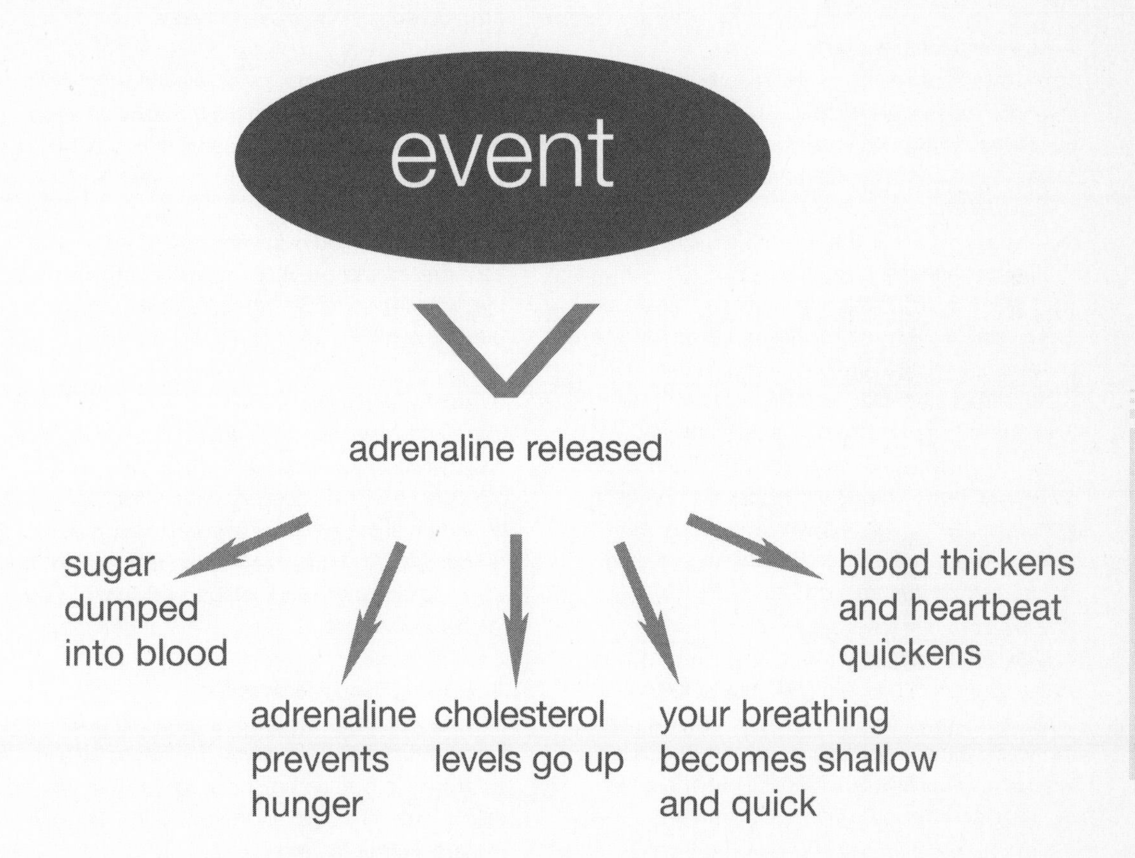

the serotonin roundabout

1 Low serotonin lifestyle

Low serotonin can make you feel sad. You may also be impulsive, have volatile reactions to moderate events and have difficulty paying attention. In the extreme, low serotonin can lead to obsession with routine or even suicidal tendencies.

2 Hunger changes

Food starts to become an important part of your day — you have cravings and can't seem to satisfy that hollow empty hunger. If you've always turned to food when feeling miserable, that lifestyle pattern will be activated at this point. You're feeling empty and search for those foods that temporarily fill you up and give you a "high." This is why people often eat fatty food when feeling low — downing the tub of ice cream is an attempt to fill the hollow empty feeling when serotonin levels are low.

3 Cravings for sugar

The changes in appetite and hunger you feel are being driven by your chemistry. Your brain is trying to manufacture more serotonin and is communicating through your appetite about what it needs but this message gets mixed up or lost in translation.

The brain searches for the protein tryptophan, which is found in dairy, meat, turkey and some nuts. This is the foundation amino acid from which serotonin is made. Your body moves this protein into the brain with the help of insulin. This process is started with the brain sending a suggestion to look for some sugar, but many sweet snacks are also high in fat and this mixture of fat and sugar doesn't do the trick. The fat slows down the insulin response and your brain doesn't get the protein it needs.

Because no serotonin is made, your cravings continue — the brain keeps sending the message for sugar and you keep eating sweet food that may or may not help the brain make serotonin.

4 Stress threshold is lowered

Your stress threshold becomes lower and events that wouldn't normally bother you now send you over the edge.

5 Apathy increases

You start to lose interest in what's going on around you. Watching your kids play in the park used to be a delight now it's drudgery, and the thought of socializing at the end of a busy week is almost unbearable. You begin to make excuses, fail to return calls and retreat into yourself, generally uninterested in what's going on.

6 Thinking becomes distorted

Your thinking becomes distorted and you personalize comments not directed at you, magnifying little things and blowing them up into major affairs. Your thinking may also become rigid and selective. You begin to mistake feelings for facts.

7 Sleep is disturbed

If you don't switch off serotonin and get some deep sleep, your brain is unable to replenish your serotonin stores throughout the night and the low serotonin cycle is perpetuated.

the serotonin roundabout

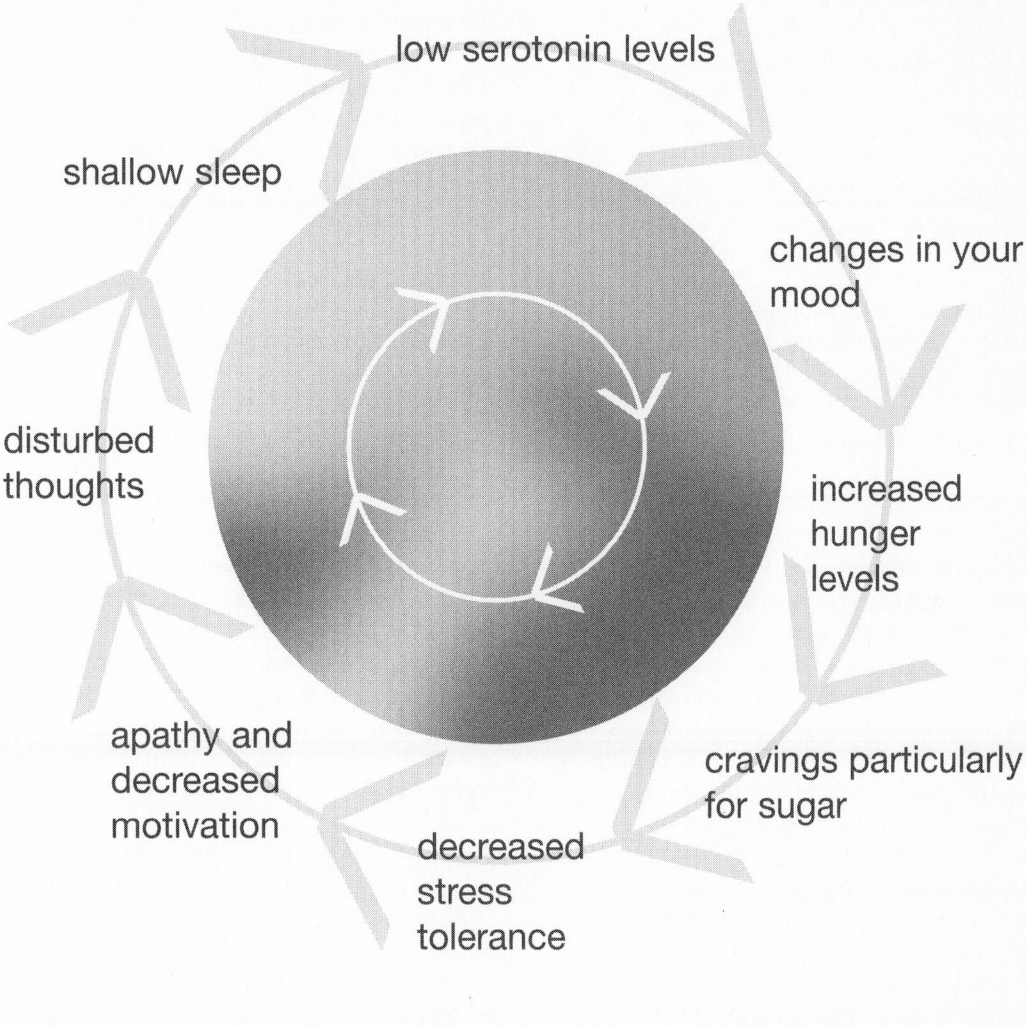

low serotonin levels

changes in your mood

increased hunger levels

cravings particularly for sugar

decreased stress tolerance

apathy and decreased motivation

disturbed thoughts

shallow sleep

the cortisol gridlock

1 High prolonged stress

When you experience a stressful event your body responds by releasing both adrenaline and cortisol. These two major players work collaboratively to manage stress events — adrenaline is the star and cortisol the understudy. With a controlled amount of stress each day, they should both work well, but constant high stress blunts the adrenaline response and increases the body's reliance on cortisol.

2 Reliance on cortisol increases

Adrenaline operates on a short-term emergency basis. Constant demands can lead to adrenaline fatigue. If this happens, cortisol begins to play a more significant part in managing the stress. Unlike adrenaline, the presence of cortisol has significant side effects including anxiety, edginess, fear or guilt.

3 Inflammation decreases

Cortisol is always accompanied by another chemical, cortisone. This has anti-inflammatory properties, its job is to reduce the swelling or damage that may occur as part of the physical response to stress. If you don't do anything to physically release your stress, it stays in your system until you can clear it. A sedentary lifestyle means cortisone and cortisol lie around causing trouble and tension.

4 Muscle tension increases

Holding you ready for fight or flight, cortisol tenses your muscles. If the stress is unrelenting you'll begin to suffer from tension headaches, a sore back and a stiff neck. If you manage to get to sleep you may wake up feeling as if you've been in a 12-round boxing bout as your joints swell and muscles ache.

5 Fat cells open

Cortisol signals the fat cells to release stored fats into the blood stream as free fatty acids. These are used as fuel for activity, once again part of the fight or flight system. If you don't metabolize them through exercising they eventually return to the fat cell for storage and the chance is gone to use up excess body fat.

6 Sugar is released

Like adrenaline, cortisol causes a blood sugar dump. The sugar is meant to help you be active in stress but if it's not used your pancreas will release insulin to lower its level. When you're active and your body is using up blood sugar for energy, the message for insulin to be released is suppressed.

This rise and then crash of blood sugar, along with the mind-altering effect of cortisol, adds to that low you get after major stress events.

7 Feelings of fear and anxiety increase

Cortisol is a mind-altering chemical. High levels for prolonged periods makes you edgy and uptight and distorts your perspective. Your tolerance decreases and you snap at those closest to you.

Sometimes this can be a useful side effect — if you're living under the fear of a stalking tiger, this heightened worry may well save your life. A little fear is healthy as it saves you from careless mistakes or from the complacency of feeling comfortable — but too much leaves you out of balance.

the cortisol gridlock

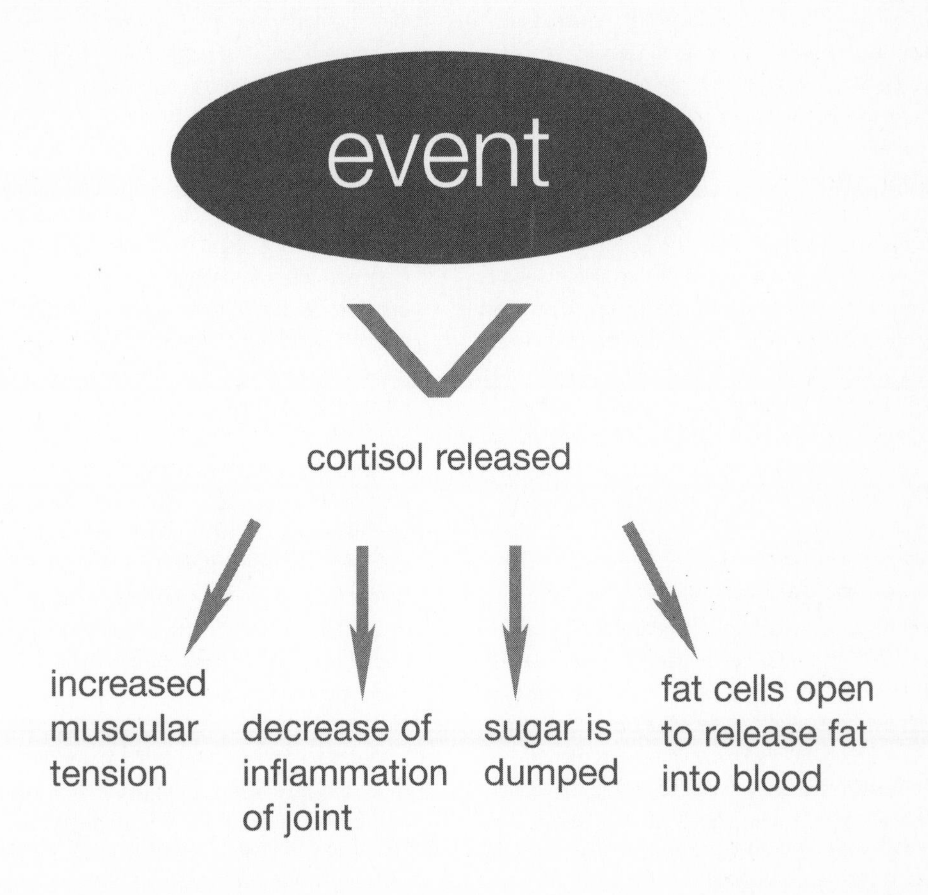

the melatonin off ramp

1 Sunlight makes melatonin

Sunlight activates the gland, deep in the brain, that manufactures the sleep chemical melatonin. Working in office buildings with artificial light hampers this system and leaving for work in the dark, eating lunch at your desk and coming home when it's dark is a recipe for insomnia.

2 Body clock is set

Your body operates on a natural rhythm determined by when you go to bed and when you get up, known as the circadian rhythm, or body clock. In the middle of the night your body temperature is low — your system starts at around 6 or 7 a.m., followed by a lowering of temperature mid afternoon with a second start up late afternoon. Inconsistent work schedules and travel that zigzags across time zones all mess with your body clock.

3 Darkness triggers melatonin

Darkness triggers melatonin and sunlight triggers serotonin. When you feel jet lagged it's because your body is trying to adjust your body clock to a new time zone, a new sleep–wake cycle. Your body gets used to these daylight and darkness times and tries to anticipate when it should switch on melatonin to sleep and serotonin to function. This is why you can often preempt an alarm clock in the morning, waking up a few minutes before it goes off.

4 Caffeine may get in the way

Caffeine remains in your system for some time after you drink it and interrupts many of the body systems designed to release melatonin and help you sleep.

5 Serotonin should switch off

Serotonin is responsible for muscle contraction — restless leg syndrome, body twitching and sleep walking are all a result of a faulty sleep–wake cycle. At night serotonin is meant to switch off so you don't act out your dreams — if for some reason your body doesn't switch off serotonin, your melatonin system can't function properly, decreasing your chances for deep restorative sleep.

6 Temperature plays a part

Body temperature also affects melatonin production. Hot summer nights of tossing and turning and sheet wrangling especially lead to frayed tempers. Sometimes your sleep partner's temperature affects your depth of sleep. Other times it's what you wear to bed or use as coverings, or the result of your fluid intake during the day.

7 Deep sleep restores body balance

A good night's sleep is the result of a well-functioning melatonin system. With a deep sleep many of the chemical imbalances created during the day are restored.

the melatonin off ramp

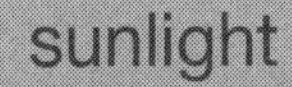

sunlight

via the eyes stimulates the pineal gland

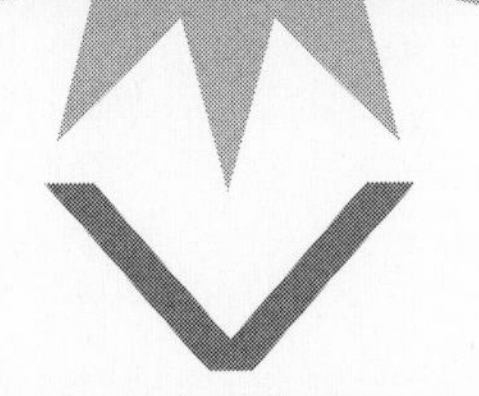

body clock is set

darkness signals the release of melatonin

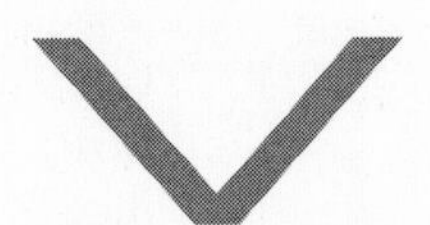

serotonin turns off

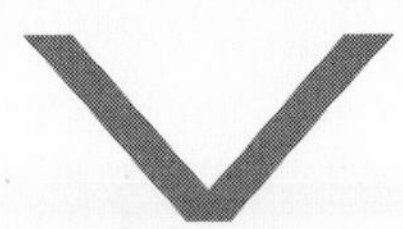

deep sleep restores chemical balance

and you drop into a deep sleep

the insulin crash zone

1 Sugar, a source of fuel

Your body uses sugar as a major fuel source. In the form of muscle glycogen, it's used when muscles contract to produce energy.

Sugar comes from food — not only the sugar you can see, but also from fruit, milk, rice, bread, potatoes and cereal. Some of these sugars are digested rapidly and enter the blood stream more quickly. Jellybeans, gummy bears and Swedish fish are some of the popular sweets that are quickly digested sugars.

2 The body selects sugar

Through an amazing early warning system the body registers high blood sugar. If you're highly active and biking in a triathlon, for example, your body will use the sugar for fuel as an immediate energy source. Sometimes, even if you're not active, you may lack energy and your body will use the sugar to give you a lift. The insulin dump is controlled by increasing your general level of activity and using up more of the sugar in your system — you don't need to ride in a triathlon to do this.

3 Insulin is released

When the sugar is not required the pancreas releases insulin, which helps the brain manufacture the happy chemical serotonin. Insulin takes the sugar and rapidly lowers it. If your body determines that the sugar is not required for activity or basic energy, it needs to remove it from your system. Small controlled doses of sugar, and the subsequent insulin reaction, cause the proteins in the blood near the blood brain barrier to clear out. This leaves two amino acids, tyrosine and tryptophan, free to cross into the brain where they in turn become dopamine (also responsible for pleasure responses) and serotonin.

High blood sugar damages the brain, which is why people with diabetes need to be so careful about the amount of refined, quickly digested sugars in their diet. If you have diabetes your pancreas doesn't effectively regulate the release of insulin — it may dump too much, or as in most cases, it doesn't respond at all and insulin needs to be administered via an injection several times a day, or orally in the form of tablets in mild cases.

4 The fat cells open

As insulin races through your system it causes the fat cells to open and push any free fatty acids in the blood inside, making room in the bloodstream for insulin to work on sugar unhindered. This is why sugar can make you fat. Not that the sugar gets forced into the fat cell but rather your fat cell becomes a fat magnet, storing every available fatty molecule in your blood. Only fat is stored in a fat cell — sugar is converted into fat via the process of lypogenesis, before it's stored.

5 Brain proteins cross over

When insulin races through the system, certain proteins are pushed into the brain. Just like fats being pushed out of the blood into the fat cell, proteins are pushed into muscle and across the blood brain barrier.

These proteins are then used to produce many useful chemicals including the happy chemical serotonin.

the insulin crash zone

eat sugar

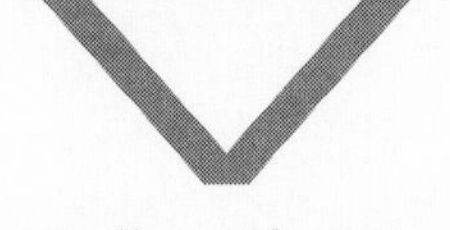

insulin released

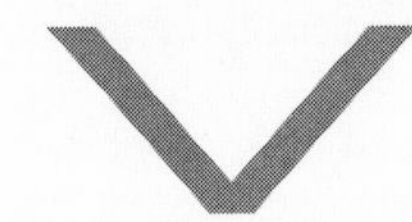

blood and brain sugar affected

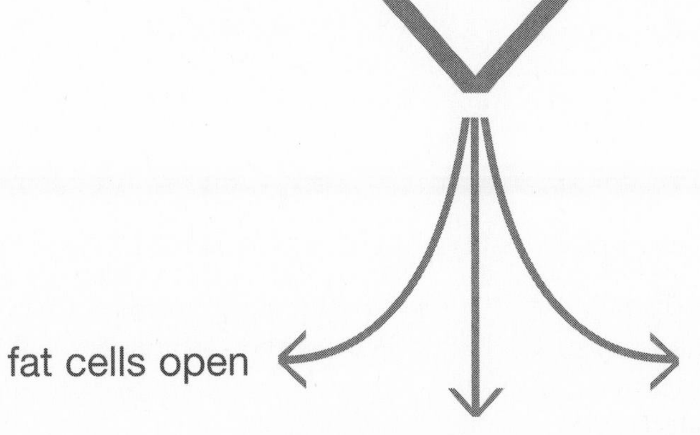

fat cells open

brain proteins cross over

cholesterol goes up

6 Cholesterol goes up

Insulin increases your cholesterol. Everyone manufactures some cholesterol and more than two thirds of the body's cholesterol is manufactured rather than eaten. If you often eat a lot of refined sugars you'll have an insulin response resulting in higher cholesterol.

Although you need to watch the amount of animal fat and refined sugar you eat, your genetic make–up also plays an important role. There are those who drink a bottle of Scotch a day, chain smoke, live on fried foods, never exercise and have low cholesterol. There are others who jog regularly, eat well and still report high cholesterol. Both of these conditions are a result of genetics — some people are programmed to have higher cholesterol and can't do much about it.

7 Blood sugar is lowered

Finally, insulin lowers your blood sugar. Your ideal blood sugar level is not always achieved — too much sugar will make you hyperactive, too little and you become drowsy and lethargic.

highways

By charting the flow of each chemical, you get an understanding of how they affect your life. Adrenaline is an expressway, powering through your body, supercharging you and setting your body up for fight or flight. Serotonin is a roundabout and affected by a number of variables, including what you eat and how you sleep. Understanding which variable needs attention in your life helps you achieve greater levels of happiness. Cortisol, melatonin and insulin also have their own unique mode of action. As you become more aware of the highways for each chemical you will see the consequences of overreliance on one or two.

1 Each of the five key chemicals in your body creates a distinct cascade of physical events and changes. By learning to recognize their effects, you can intervene in the process and take better control of your moods. You can choose a lifestyle that balances your chemistry and leads to a calmer, more productive life.

2 The process of adrenaline is similar to a highway. It moves at high speed in one direction and leads to dramatic wholesale changes in how you feel and operate. You may also be heading in a direction that doesn't take you exactly to your goal and sometimes you're just going so fast you miss the turn off. There's also the potential for high speed crashes.

3 The process of serotonin is similar to a roundabout. Each event leads to the next and it's often hard to determine which part of the cycle is causing the problem. Each step in the process is a way into the cycle — your sleep loss may be affecting the process or it may be what you eat or how you think. When things are not working well, you feel like you're driving the wrong way on the roundabout, experiencing a series of near misses and high anxiety.

4 The process of cortisol is like an impatient driver in gridlock — your blood boils over, you honk the horn, pull out and work the accelerator and brake hard. Like the wear and tear on the car, cortisol gridlock burns you out and wears you down. You may even have accidents with the people nearest to you even though they're not responsible for the traffic jam.

5 The process of melatonin is like an off ramp. If you find a way to locate the off ramp you can normally take a rest from the hustle and bustle of life and reenter the highway after a break, refueled and with a better sense for whether you're heading in the right direction. Stop, revive survive.

lights

6 The process of insulin is like a crash zone. All other traffic slows down, while insulin rushes though your system like paramedics in an ambulance. You have to pull over and rest for a while and let the insulin do its job. Only when the crash has been cleaned up does the traffic begin to flow again.

Manners require time.

As nothing is more vulgar than haste.

RALPH WALDO EMERSON

3

adrenaline junkies

YOU KNOW YOU'RE AN ADRENALINE JUNKIE WHEN INSTANT COFFEE ISN'T FAST ENOUGH; YOU READ FAXES AS THEY COME IN; YOU NEED DEADLINES TO GET ANYTHING DONE; AND YOU'VE FORGOTTEN HOW TO RELAX.

all fired up

For as long as I can remember I've loved being busy. I seem to always need something to do and never wanted to just sit around — even as a child I would eat lunch up a tree and read on the bus on the way home! Now I carry extra work to meetings in case people are late and my vacation itineraries require a full time manager. I can't imagine being without my Day Planner. I drive to the gym with the radio on; run on the treadmill with a favorite CD and then arrive home to watch my favorite shows pre-recorded so I can fast forward the ads. In fact, I think I fast forward everything. Often I fall asleep in front of the TV only to wake up a few hours later, trudge up the hall and flop into bed. I have begun to use delays as a chance to think about my goals and have booked a vacation with no plans. I still record my favorite shows and fast forward the ads — some things just make sense!

If you've ever fallen asleep at the wheel of your car on a long drive, you recognize adrenaline as that "rush" that courses through your system when you snap awake to find yourself swerving across the road. It's the same thing that speeds up your heart rate before you even take your first step on a run. It's released into your system when a nightmare wakes you, sweating and flinching. Adrenaline also speeds up your heart rate when you see someone you're attracted to.

Because adrenaline is the rush chemical it makes you think fast, talk rapidly and want everything around you to hurry up. A crammed life is typical of the adrenaline junkie — you try to be "on" 100% of the time. If you've been doing this for some time, you'll literally be addicted to the "rush" and may have lost the ability to relax. But even though there's a direct parallel between adrenaline addiction and stress illness, you probably don't think of yourself as stressed. In your mind, you're simply going fast in a stressed-out world.

When you learn to switch onto adrenaline only when you need to, and manage the rush in a healthy, balanced way, you can be naturally high more often, rather than using your "drug" to get through everyday life.

are you at risk of adrenaline addiction?

Score description

0 This statement does not apply to me.
1 This statement applies to me (say less than once a month).
2 This statement often applies to me (say more than once a month).

1 I feel as if there isn't enough time in each day to do all the things I need to do.

2 I speak more quickly than other people, even finishing their sentences for them.

3 My relatives and friends say, or I believe, that I eat too quickly.

4 I would rather win than enjoy a game.

5 I am very competitive at work, sport or games.

6 I tend to be bossy and dominate others.

7 I prefer to lead than follow.

8 I feel pressed for time even when I'm not doing something important.

9 I become more impatient when I have to wait for something or when I'm interrupted.

10 I tend to make decisions quickly and compulsively.

11 I take on more than I can accomplish.

12 I become irritable (and even angry) more often than other people.

13 I often feel a strong compulsion to be doing something while at home or on vacation.

14 I fidget often or become restless — pacing, leg kicking or fast gum chewing.

15 I get a vague feeling of depression whenever I stop an activity.

Total score

Out of a possible score of 30 you would have fallen into one of the following four categories:

0-10	Relaxed
10-15	Typical
15-20	On the edge
20+	Adrenaline junkie

quiz

SNAPSHOT

The feeling of adrenaline in your system is addictive.

A reliance on adrenaline to be naturally high is not good for serotonin levels.

Your body often uses cortisol when you don't have enough adrenaline to meet stress demands.

If you sleep well and maintain melatonin levels you can survive being an adrenaline junkie.

Because adrenaline dumps sugar into your system you may suffer from an insulin overreaction.

There's no right or wrong answer to the adrenaline addiction questionnaire. It's simply a tool to identify whether you sit on the relaxed or the stimulated side of the spectrum. Everyone uses adrenaline to get through tough parts of the day, but if you have a high score you're trying to run on adrenaline all the time — a situation that will only lead to burnout and exhaustion. By being constantly on adrenaline you end up crashing more often than if you made use of your other body chemistry. You may also need help controlling your adrenaline when you're "on."

Personality profile tests group people into two general categories: type A and type B. A type A personality is the classic workaholic, highly strung "I don't have time for this meeting" person. Type B is characterized by the relaxed, laid-back individual who is likely to have so much time up their sleeve they won't even turn up for the meeting.

You'll often see people at the top of the corporate tree showing both type A and B character traits. A study in a *Harvard Business Review* special report found that the ability to stay calm in crisis was one of the most prized character traits for leaders today. At the same time, anyone who can't get passionate or committed to what they're doing is likely to fail in today's highly competitive world. It's about balance.

side effects of 100% adrenaline

If you're trying to be "on" 100% of the time, you're in danger of abusing adrenaline and ultimately crashing.

Sick on stopping

You slow down and get sick. This is because high adrenaline falsely maintains your immune system —

for a while. When you eventually crash down off the adrenaline you have a lowered immune system and so are more likely to catch a cold.

Vacation crash

For the first couple of days when you go on vacation you crash in a heap, unable to lift a finger for any activity other than saying "Bartender — another margarita!" A few days into your vacation you regret the choice of an isolated island retreat because there "just isn't anything to do here!" Being used to over-stimulation you find it hard to idle. You only know two speeds: "on" or "crashed."

Saturday sleep-in

You wake up at your usual time of 7:00 a.m. on a Saturday morning, only to realize it's the weekend, so you go back to bed. Two hours later you wake up feeling worse than if you'd gotten up at 7:00. This is either because you've interrupted a typical sleep cycle of 90 minutes, or because your body has begun to unwind and come off adrenaline — a mini crash. Often it's a mixture of both.

Artificial deadlines

You always wait until the last minute to get anything done, at which point you have no choice but to work late to finish your work. Alternatively, you create a false sense of urgency with artificial deadlines so that you get working on a project before the deadline. But creating a sense of urgency is only useful if you're lacking motivation and need to get going on a difficult task.

Long weekend dreams

Saturday you wake up restless; so you get up, wash the car, do some gardening, clean the house, take the kids to play football and get home Saturday afternoon hoping to read the weekend paper. You get halfway through the front page and fall asleep on the sofa.

Your partner wakes you, reminding you to get ready for a dinner party with friends. You don't know why, but the idea of light conversation feels too much like hard work. You go to the party and, after a drink or two, unwind and begin to enjoy the night. Sunday morning you feel less restless than the day before. You relax into the family barbecue at lunch and by Sunday night you're beginning to feel normal again. You know that if you had one more relaxed day you might actually begin to feel human again. (If this is you, you may not be a complete junkie yet, but you're getting close!)

the adrenaline crash

As a professional speaker, I'm in front of an audience an average of three times a week. Each time I give a workshop I switch into my adrenaline system so that I can present with the energy and enthusiasm required. I get into a state of arousal and readiness. When it fires, I have a great time, but afterward, there's the danger of a crash. To minimize the crash I go back to my room, close the door, run a bath (regardless of the time of day) and chill for about 20 minutes. I then get dressed slowly and methodically go about checking out. The key is avoiding the temptation to rush into something else and stay "on stage."

Because the adrenaline high state is addictive, you may be trying to be "on" 100% of the time. The end result is a heavy crash — you get home at the end of a day's work and have no time or energy for "life."

Do you have adrenaline withdrawal?

1 Do you have a strong compulsion to be doing something else while at home or on vacation?
2 Are you obsessed with thoughts about what remains undone?
3 Do you have a vague feeling of guilt when relaxing?
4 Do you fidget and suffer from restlessness, pacing, leg kicking and fast gum chewing?
5 Do you have a vague feeling of depression or anticlimax?

You will have felt the adrenaline crash after the completion of a major project — instead of being elated you find yourself walking around feeling empty and hollow. To avoid the crash, and reduce the roller-coaster effect, you need to manage your ups and downs more effectively. You'll stay high more often if you learn how to improve the balance of your current chemical profile — although you may crash coming off adrenaline, high levels of serotonin cushion the fall.

making adrenaline work for you

On adrenaline

The key to being naturally high 80% of the time and "up" when you need to be, is knowing when a push of adrenaline is required and when you need to conserve it. It's the prolonged abuse of adrenaline that leaves some people burned out rather than fired up.

Most people don't need to boost their adrenaline levels — nature will switch it on at times of need. But you do need to have laid a good foundation by ensuring your serotonin system is functioning, then make sure you don't exhaust your adrenaline system through overuse. Although caffeine and other drugs, fatty foods, pressure and "pep talks" can all trigger adrenaline release, if everything else is working well, you'll rarely need to deliberately stimulate adrenaline in your system — when the time comes it will be there.

Go APE

While "losing it" is not usually a good idea, there are times in your life when you need to put in a big effort and go APE. These are Adrenaline Priority Events, moments when you need to dig in and get on with the task, when you should go fast, think quickly and make rapid decisions. If you have a crisis and you need to use adrenaline, go for it! Deadlines, emergencies at work and important projects require a certain push. Adrenaline, and what it provides, help you through these times. You're in crisis mode, so do the best you can, tap your adrenaline system and work it out.

Do you need to slow down?

1 How could you enjoy more pause in your life?

2 Are you allowing time for your body to tell you what it needs?

3 If you're running fast all the time is there something you're avoiding?

4 What can you eliminate from your life so you can spend more time doing what you want to?

Look at your day in advance and choose when you think Adrenaline Priority Events are likely to occur. Then spend the rest of the day sparing adrenaline for those moments. By doing this you can manage hours of stress a day and still go home calm and relaxed. But always remember, you can only do this for so many hours a day before cortisol kicks in and you get uptight and stressed out.

Slow down

If you do everything in fast forward you need to step off speed and make some space in your life.

When you leave work, drive in silence or come prepared to read on the bus or listen to a CD. Then read for an hour or so when you get home before you switch on the TV. If you find yourself nodding off, go to bed a little earlier — you'll sleep through the night more often. You may still want to watch an hour or so of TV after reading, but the initial pause from TV's stimulation is just enough for your body to tell you of its need for sleep.

If you're coming home to a rush hour with kids, try to take a moment for yourself earlier in the day. Often when the kids are asleep or at school you go into a powerhouse mode and get everything done that you can't do when they're around. This should include enjoying a moment of calm on the couch.

One of the fundamental rules of growth is to pause after activity allowing yourself to absorb the lesson or adjust to the new knowledge. Body builders also use a day of rest after each workout to ensure the muscle cells adapt to the training session. If you're an adrenaline junkie, sitting on a park bench and doing nothing is totally foreign to you, so make sure you schedule some time when you do absolutely nothing.

giving yourself a boost

Even if you're the most addicted adrenaline junkie you'll have flat days and from time to time you need to juice up your adrenal system to get a jolt of motivation. While purposely hyping up your system is the worst thing you can do if you're stressed or burned out, a little kick-start can help one of those slow days. So if you need to push a natural high, try one of the following strategies.

Caffeine

A cup of coffee (which acts directly on your adrenal system) in the morning will give your day a running start. Caffeine is a drug and like most drugs, problems occur when you abuse the amount you have. The average human can handle 300 mg (about five cups, depending on the way the coffee is prepared) maximum caffeine per day without negative side effects. If you drink more than this you'll become habituated and will start experiencing dramatic side effects such as headaches, dehydration and nervous system problems. It's wise to drink fewer than five cups a day and also have some coffee-free days.

Fatty food

High fat foods give your adrenal system a temporary spike. If you're under pressure you probably turn to red meat, whole milk dairy foods and nuts. While this seems like a good idea at the time, more often than not it causes an uncontrolled response, leaving you feeling lethargic and in a low performance state. What you really need to do under pressure is eat more vegetables, fish and skinless chicken, as this boosts more supportive brain chemistry.

Artificial deadlines

Some time management schools suggest you create a sense of urgency if you need to get things done. If you're an adrenaline junkie you use harsh self-talk and artificial deadlines to keep yourself on an adrenaline high. Adrenaline is your "fight or flight" chemical, so if you think it's warranted, playing mental games with yourself to force action may be useful as a stick and carrot form of motivation. Although this may work in the short term, getting your goals and passions in alignment so that your motivation becomes intrinsic and less reliant on outside factors is a better strategy.

Motivational seminars, pep talks and religious rallies

For some, a quick way to achieve an adrenaline high is to attend mass gatherings or receive emotional pep talks to get "fire in the belly." Successful sporting team coaches will often, at half-time, rev up players with a fiery speech about what it means to get out on the field and win. If the focus of your motivation is short term, this quick hit strategy works well — enduring motivation needs more than fire and heat. Although true change requires a constant application of effort, the "pep talk" approach is probably the healthiest alternative for kicking in your adrenaline — it's not a drug (so has no side effects) and is positively centered (rather than pressure centered like artificial deadlines).

adrenaline junkies

While adrenaline gives you a rush and allows you to be highly productive, you can't run on it all day. Going at everything 100 miles an hour (typical of an adrenaline junkie) leads to adrenal fatigue. A constant use of the adrenaline emergency system results in stress as the body struggles to meet the high pressure needs 24 hours a day 7 days a week. Choosing adrenaline moments by slowing down everyday activities and focusing adrenaline energy where it will do the most good will lead to a naturally high life.

The problem with abusing adrenaline is the risk of burnout.
Are you a candidate for the burn?

1 Do you feel let down by the people around you? ❍ yes ❍ no
2 Are you too busy for close friends and family? ❍ yes ❍ no
3 Are you too busy to do even routine things like send out thank you notes, return phone calls or mail birthday cards? ❍ yes ❍ no
4 Do you tire more easily than you used to? ❍ yes ❍ no
5 Are you working harder but accomplishing less? ❍ yes ❍ no
6 Are you increasingly cynical and disenchanted? ❍ yes ❍ no
7 Are you often invaded by a sadness you can't explain? ❍ yes ❍ no
8 Do you forget appointments, deadlines, possessions? ❍ yes ❍ no
9 Are you increasingly irritable? More short tempered? ❍ yes ❍ no
10 Does your body ache or are you having trouble shaking a cold? ❍ yes ❍ no
11 Are you finding it harder to be happy and joyful? ❍ yes ❍ no
12 Have you lost your sense of humor? ❍ yes ❍ no
13 Have you lost interest in sex? ❍ yes ❍ no
14 Are you less talkative than you used to be? ❍ yes ❍ no

TOTAL (add up your yes answers) ❑ yes ❑ no

Your score

0-5	Cruising along nicely
5-10	Borderline burnout
10-15	Burnout candidate

This is one quiz in which a low score is good. If you score under 5, you are handling your stress well and are most likely to be balancing your body chemistry. If you scored between 5 and 10, you are a burnout candidate. Be wary of taking on new work or extra commitments if you know you are already spread thin. Factor in a little personal time and check your priorities. If you scored higher than 10, you need to take immediate steps to avoid a crash. Write a list of what's important in your day, and eliminate activities that don't support your main goals. Identify what you need to get rid of and ask yourself what you are wasting time on.

1 The adrenaline-based “rush” state is a peak performance state. The key to using it well is to only use it at appropriate times. Many people who lead high-pressure lifestyles become addicted to the rush feeling — a literal addiction to adrenaline.

2 Relaxation when peak performance is required is not the answer. Holding the aroused state when it’s needed, then letting go of it when it’s not, is the key.

3 Coming out of the adrenaline rush is often experienced as a crash — like coming off an artificial drug. High serotonin levels and practice make this process gentler and faster.

highlights

4 Caffeine and other drugs, fatty foods, pressure and “pep talks” can all trigger adrenaline release. But, if everything else is working well, it’s rarely necessary to deliberately stimulate adrenaline in your system.

Happiness makes up in

height for what it lacks in length.

ROBERT FROST

4

serotonin seekers

YOU KNOW YOU'RE A SEROTONIN SEEKER WHEN A SUNNY DAY MAKES YOU HAPPY, YOU CRAVE SUGAR MID AFTERNOON AND A MASSAGE RATES AS ONE OF LIFE'S GREATEST PLEASURES.

the sustainable natural high

I love the constant pressure of my job although it hasn't always been that way. I used to think I wasn't cut out for it — many of the people I worked with seemed to be better set up for the high pressure. They matched stress with high energy and as the work got tougher they got louder and faster. It was only after I'd been working there for some time that I noticed a lot of them had left — they burned out. I went through a stage when I thought the pressure would kill me, but one day it hit me when I was sitting in the lunch room and looking back into the office. The lunch room was pristine, not a dirty plate anywhere. No one else on the whole floor had stopped to have something to eat. Now I won't miss a meal, I exercise outside every day and get a massage once a week. I truly believe that eating, exercising and being touched keep me going in an industry when most burn out by the time they're 30.

Adrenaline junkies are focused on productivity and eliminating stress, serotonin seekers are chasing happiness. When you have enough serotonin you're happy, calm, comfortable and satisfied. Not enough and you're depressed, moody, stressed, guilty and inclined to put on weight.

If you're a serotonin seeker you'll spend a great deal of time in your head — adrenaline junkies may act without thinking, serotonin seekers often think without acting. While the adrenaline high is exciting, it's not long lasting — a well functioning serotonin system will help you manage your adrenaline so that you can use it to its best advantage.

The drug of optimism and happiness, serotonin makes you joyful and more generous of spirit. It also has many other enduring psychological and physical benefits.

Calm decision making

If you have adequate levels of serotonin, you're calmer and more self-assured. You'll be able to handle change and pressure well with a serotonin high. But when serotonin is low your perceptions become distorted, you're more likely to be confused and unable to think through problems.

Creativity and innovation

It's hard to be creative when you're depressed. To be innovative you need a serotonin high and not enough serotonin is responsible for most depression.

Head monkey

The head monkey in every group is the one with the highest serotonin. Those monkeys lower in status and with low serotonin act out, becoming angry and violent. In time they can become outcasts, with last pick of a mate and often missing out on their share of the group meal.

Less impulsive

With a serotonin high you'll be more in control and less impulsive. Children who are aggressive and antisocial have been shown to have low serotonin levels. Impulsive violent offenders also have low serotonin levels, including those who use extreme forms of violence against others.

Weight control

Whether you feel full or not depends greatly on serotonin. When you're full or satisfied, serotonin (along with other chemicals) sends a message via the hypothalamus that you're done. If your serotonin system doesn't function properly this message doesn't get through and you overeat.

Fewer cravings

Food and mood are closely linked. If you're on a serotonin low your brain will desperately try to correct the imbalance and create a natural high. It does this by firing off the chemical responsible for food cravings, particularly those high in sugar.

Better circulation

Some drugs prescribed for heart conditions work on serotonin and its active partners. Through the blood, serotonin helps heal wounds and works on blood vessels, opening and closing them as required.

Fewer headaches

Some people who have taken antidepressants have reported an easing of tension or migraine headaches. Although it doesn't work in everyone, it's believed that

SNAPSHOT

A reliance on adrenaline to feel great can lower serotonin.

High serotonin is the key to enduring motivation.

Cortisol leaves little room for serotonin to work its magic.

Melatonin at night is needed for deep sleep and good supplies of serotonin on waking.

Insulin and sugar are key to serotonin production.

desperately seeking serotonin

Score description

0 This statement does not apply to me.
1 This statement applies to me (say less than once a month).
2 This statement often applies to me (say more than once a month).

1 I gain weight quickly when I stop dieting.

2 I notice that the seasons affect my mood, particularly winter or overcast days.

3 Some days I feel a profound sadness for no reason.

4 I tend to eat when I'm unhappy or after I have had an argument.

5 I feel like I live two lives; one in my head and one in my actual life.

6 In the afternoon all I can think of is my next sugar hit.

7 Often, after completing a major project I have a hollow empty feeling.

8 I find it hard to concentrate in meetings if I am not asked to contribute.

9 I often eat food straight from the container while standing.

10 Sometimes I eat without even being conscious that I am eating; often I can't even remember what I ate.

11 I can't even bring myself to answer a phone call from my best friend.

12 I have trouble collecting my thoughts, particularly in the afternoons.

13 I tend to create problem situations before they even exist.

14 I eat when I am bored.

15 I am often tired but unable to get to sleep.

Total score

So how did you rate? Out of a possible score of 30 you would have fallen into one of the following four categories:

0-10	Serotonin not a concern
10-15	Normal serotonin challenges
15-20	Borderline seeker
20+	Serotonin seeker

in some cases it's due to the vasoconstriction (shrinking) effect serotonin has on the blood vessels that dilate (expand) in tension headaches.

Better muscle control

Serotonin is crucial to muscle contraction. Sleepwalking and restless leg syndrome are caused by a dysfunctional sleep–wake cycle — your body forgets to turn off serotonin and so you contract your muscles and move about in your sleep.

young brains

If you were born in 1900 you would have had a life expectancy of just 50 years. Today it lies somewhere between 75 and 85 years with an increasing number of people living well past 90. Having identified the gene responsible for aging, scientists at the Human Genome Project are predicting many people born in the near future will live well beyond 100. So it's important your mental faculties keep up with the increasing life expectancy — preserving serotonin levels will encourage mental longevity to accompany extended biological aging.

Low levels of serotonin have specifically been linked to those with Alzheimer's disease, and aggressive and impulsive behavior sometimes associated with Alzheimer's has been successfully treated with antidepressant medication. Caregivers in nursing home facilities have also observed at sunset that many residents become disoriented and sometimes aggressive. Known as sundowning, preliminary research attributes this to the poor lighting in many homes and the residents' lack of sunlight during the day. The pineal gland also produces less melatonin in older people making sleep less effective. These factors combine to create a confused sleep–wake cycle in those who suffer from sundowning. Although the solution isn't simple, many carers of the aged are placing residents outside in the sun more often, brightening up the rooms and halls and also introducing exercise programs to increase melatonin production.

SAD vacation

I was in Europe, the dream vacation of a lifetime. I should have had a ball. At first when I felt so depressed I thought it was just jet lag, but after a few weeks I began to think it was something more. The weather wasn't marvelous; the sky was gray almost every day. I had imagined this holiday in my mind for so many years — the wonderful art galleries and the feeling of so much history to be enjoyed. Yet, there I was, feeling so low, asking myself, "What's wrong with me?"

The second leg of the tour was much better as we headed for sunnier climes. This was the leg of the tour where we all recovered, lying around on chairs by the pool, sipping the exotic drink of the day and soaking up a little sunshine. I began to feel like my old self again after a few days — I started to wonder if the jet lag, my tiredness and the bad weather had all combined to knock me about.

Researchers at the National Institute for Mental Health have found links between low serotonin and seasonal affective disorder syndrome (SADS). SADS often occurs in countries with few daylight hours — by not getting enough daylight, people become depressed. Using light boxes, specially designed solariums, the people who suffered from SADS were able to improve their moods considerably. The link is still not clear but probably has to do with the relationship between exposure to sunlight and the pineal gland. Located in the middle of your brain this tiny pea- like gland manufactures the sleep drug melatonin and is sensitive to daylight. Because serotonin and melatonin work hand in hand, they ensure you sleep when you should (melatonin) and that you wake and move when you need to (serotonin).

obsessions

Characterized by ritual repetitive movements, Obsessive Compulsive Disorder (OCD) encompasses a wide spectrum of intensities, from counting your steps as you walk down a certain street to counting the number of cornflakes in your cereal bowl. While OCD is complex behavior, there are certain obvious links to a serotonin imbalance and it's often treated with antidepressant medications that act on the serotonin system.

One study at Princeton University using cats found that the repetitive grooming techniques were a form of self medication. They drew the conclusion that people with OCD may be doing the same thing when they wash their hands 20 times in an hour or chew gum relentlessly. Low levels of serotonin fuel anxiety and your anxiety rituals may be indicative of a serotonin seeker's profile.

happy brains

The key to increasing serotonin in your brain and achieving a natural high is to adjust your lifestyle.

Eat more meat

Turkey, red meat and almonds are just a few of the foods rich in tryptophan, the basic protein from which your brain manufactures serotonin. Eating these every other day ensures you have enough protein available for the brain to manufacture happy drugs.

For the brain to have access to these building blocks you need to clear the blood around the brain with a controlled sugar hit — but most people overdose on the sugar in response to the craving and end up asleep or lacking energy as insulin rages through their system in response to the huge sugar dump. If you eat foods rich in tryptophan, then each day have a controlled sugar hit and wait 20 minutes for the serotonin to kick in. Ideal hits include 1/3 cup of raisins or two bananas.

Allow time to recover

Program some pause into your day and identify how often you need that pause. Some people need a break every hour, others can work flat out for a week before they need to rest. Some people choose occupations where they can go for six months without a break and then take the rest of the year off. You need a balance of hard and easy, fast and slow, so your body can rebalance its chemistry in the rest periods.

Get outside

If you have a profile that includes serotonin, you will gain great benefit from being outdoors. Eat your lunch

Need some help cheering up? Ask yourself these questions.

1. What could I do to get more sunshine in my day?
2. How can I eat more vegetables, turkey, almonds and red meat?
3. How can I make my sleep more effective? Could I go to bed and get up at the same time each day?
4. How do I think? Am I negative in my self-talk? What could I do about changing this?
5. What habits have I developed around eating? Do I eat when I'm bored? Do I eat when I have a cup of tea?

outside, not at your desk and have breakfast on the back porch rather than in the kitchen. Exercise at lunchtime with a walk in the park. When the smokers in your office go outside for a cigarette, you can go for a sunshine/serotonin hit — even an overcast day will create a better chemical balance profile than a whole day spent under fluorescent lighting.

Adopt regular sleeping habits

Deep sleep gives your body time to generate serotonin and rebalance your daily chemical use. Go to bed and get up at set times so your body learns when it should manufacture your sleep drug melatonin and when it should switch on serotonin. Avoid making radical changes to your sleep pattern and don't sleep in — that feeling of lethargy many people feel at the start of the working week ("Monday-i-tis") is caused by the weekend sleep-in.

Get touched regularly

If you're not being touched regularly, why not pay for a professional massage? Therapeutic massage has been shown to have a positive effect on those with mild depression. Babies who are massaged as infants also show greater independence, confidence and mental resilience.

Pets can also be good therapy. Throughout the United States, hospitals, nursing homes and mental healthcare facilities are just some of the settings where "therapy pets" (most often cats and dogs) are providing the therapeutic benefits of unconditional love and physical contact to children and adults.

Do easy exercise

There has been some evidence that easy exercise elevates serotonin and decreases depression. This means working out every other day, going for a walk, swimming some laps, playing with the dog or hitting a round of golf. The human body was made to move and the dramatic decrease in physical activity in the past few decades is causing severe chemical imbalances.

extra help for depression

I used to wake up every morning not wanting to start another day. This is the "dark cloud" of depression — it doesn't matter what causes it, the devastating effect is the same. I simply didn't want to go on living. Often I would get panic attacks and it was hard to imagine that life would ever hold any joy again.

A friend, who had also lost a child told me, "Happy times will come again." At the time I found this hard to grasp, but looking back, I realize he was right. We have to be aware of the disabling effect of depression on our lives and take all the positive steps available to combat this very crippling condition. Antidepressants gave me the edge to cope — I don't need them any more but at the time who knows what I might have done.

Many people with low serotonin need to restore the chemical imbalance that leads to depression and need to do so quickly. This is where antidepressants, whether prescription or herbal, may help.

If you're very depressed and think you could benefit from antidepressants, talk to your doctor about the new generation of less severe SSRI (selective serotonin reuptake inhibitors) antidepressants, such as Prozac and Zoloft, which act on the receptor site between the brain cells where serotonin exists. If you're suffering from depression, the serotonin levels in this gap are low and so the connection that would increase happiness and stabilize mood is unable to function properly — the message doesn't get through.

Serotonin is released and returned from different parts of the brain cell. The SSRI antidepressants act as locks at the site where serotonin is returned. This prevents the nerve cell from reabsorbing the serotonin already in circulation. After a few weeks on antidepressants your levels of serotonin build up and the message they convey becomes stronger. This allows the "happy" connection caused by serotonin to stay "on" for longer, allowing you to cope better with your life.

Although SSRI antidepressants reportedly have fewer side effects than their predecessor (monoamine oxidase inhibitors or MAOIs), you may still find you have decreased libido, weight gain, headaches and drowsiness to name a few of the side effects.

The most common of the herbal over–the–counter antidepressants, St. John's wort and hypericum, have been shown to have a positive effect on mild depression. Hypericum in particular has been used to treat SADS.

Some people taking hypericum do get sensitivity to the sun, so if you're already suffering from sun-related skin conditions you need to be careful taking it. It's also important not to mix hypericum and St. John's wort with prescribed medication, including anti-depressants, as this can cause major disturbances in the effect of the prescribed drugs and is particularly dangerous without medical supervision.

The over-the-counter herbal antidepressant 5-htp has been shown in preliminary studies to be as effective as hypericum or St. John's wort. Many people prefer it to herbs because it mimics the actual substance 5-htp in your body (food such as almonds turn into tryptophan, which becomes 5-htp and then crosses the blood brain barrier, finally being used to create serotonin).

Despite limited research to date, two other non-prescription options for dealing with depression, SAM-e (s-adenosylemethionine) and TMG (trimethyl-glycine), have shown promising results. Both drugs act at different stages of neurotransmitter manufacture. Doctors in the UK have been recommending SAM-e

how antidepressants work

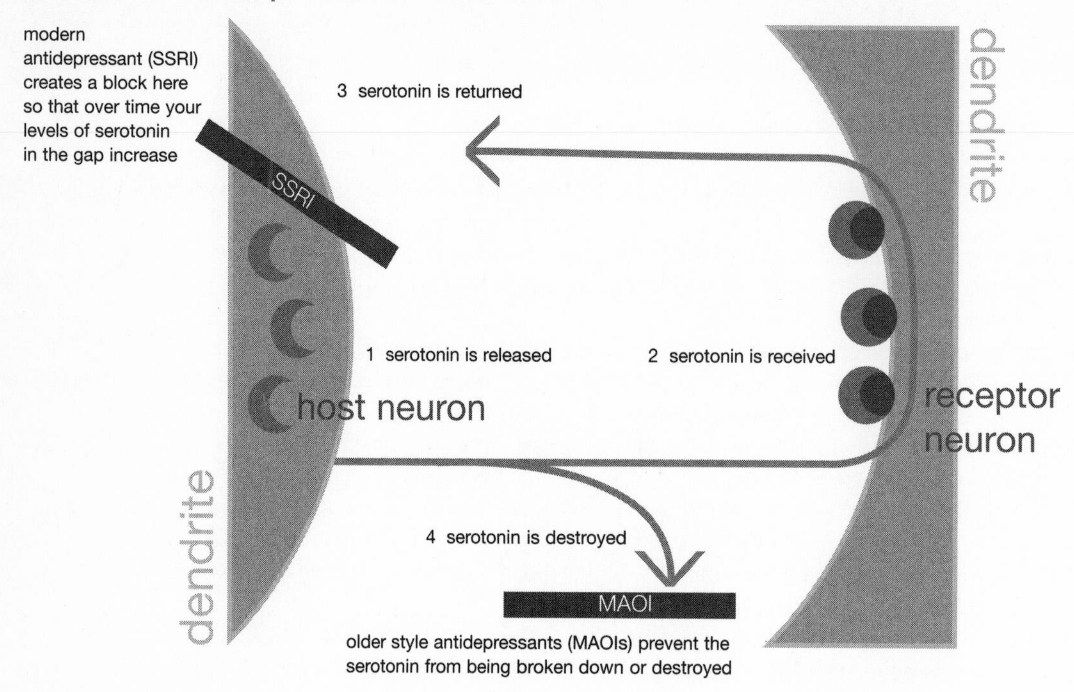

as an alternative to antidepressants in cases of mild to moderate depression for over 10 years. Both drugs appear to be most effective if combined with B vitamins and if taken before eating. If your doctor is not familiar with SAM-e and TMG talk to a naturopath. He or she will advise you on dosages and what to eat.

If you're feeling low and decide to treat yourself with herbal antidepressants, monitor yourself closely as self-medication often leaves a major condition untreated that may worsen if left alone.

serotonin seekers

Serotonin provides a calm enduring alternative for being fired up on adrenaline. It also controls appetite and regulates many daily functions including memory. Sleep, sun and sugar are key lifestyle factors that increase serotonin levels.

1 Serotonin is responsible for a range of behaviors and feelings. Too little will make you feel unhappy or depressed. With optimal levels of serotonin you're happy, calm, comfortable and satisfied.

2 Most people can create enduring motivation and lasting happiness by learning how to naturally elevate serotonin levels.

3 Impulsive, obsessive or aggressive behavior is a warning sign indicating lowered serotonin levels.

4 Antidepressant medication works in many cases to counter a low serotonin genetic make-up.

5 SSRI antidepressants such as Prozac and Zoloft act on your brain cells to elevate the amount of serotonin in the synapse or gap between neurons.

lights

6 St. John's wort, 5-HTP and hypericum are all over-the-counter supplements that have been shown to counter mild depression. Don't use these if you are on any medication and always check with your doctor first.

Cocaine is just God's way of telling you you're making too much money.

ROBIN WILLIAMS

5

unnatural high

messed up highs

There are many ways to get high — both natural and unnatural. Whether you think of a drug as being natural or unnatural will depend on your personal beliefs as well as social convention. But regardless of personal or moral beliefs, or social convention, there is no doubt that drugs mess with your body's own natural chemicals and can prevent you from experiencing the wonderful natural process of feeling happy. Using drugs often suppresses your own natural "uppers" as the fast-acting, hard-hitting manufactured chemicals in drugs can lower your brain's supply of natural feel good chemicals such as serotonin and adrenaline.

Illicit drugs, including cocaine, amphetamines, heroin and crack seriously mess with your body chemistry. Because it's legal and many people smoke, tobacco is considered a lesser harm. But nicotine is addictive and definitely messes with your body chemistry.

Although drinking a little alcohol will make you feel high, if you drink too much you begin to feel low — abuse of alcohol has also destroyed many lives. Most people don't think of caffeine, which also changes your chemistry, as a drug and use it get a lift throughout the day.

illicit drugs

I had no idea what was going on with Clive. We had known each other for about 10 years and were close friends. Then we started to have unsettling get-togethers. One day he became weird after a cup of coffee — kind of punch drunk — and I had to help him across the road. At first I chalked it up to his huge success — he had everything ahead of him. Or so I thought. Because I've never been into illicit drugs it never even crossed my mind that this might be the reason for his behavior. It turned out Clive had been

SNAPSHOT

Many illicit drugs mimic or stimulate the adrenal system.

Serotonin is affected by prolonged use of marijuana and other illicit drugs.

Cortisol is affected by caffeine and alcohol.

Melatonin is affected by caffeine as the caffeine prevents sleep.

Insulin is affected by alcohol.

experimenting with all the trendy illicit drugs, from ecstasy to cocaine. He was living in the fast lane.

The giveaway for me was when he was coming off the drugs. He had always been a hyper person so the moody depression when he came down off the drugs was so out of character. From my point of view the high just wasn't worth the lows. I broached the topic with him a few times and I guess this drove us apart.

Illicit drugs will give you the most unnatural of unnatural highs. Some people feel they're not getting enough of what they seek in life so turn to these drugs to super boost their body chemistry. Many stars who are wealthy and famous often turn to illicit drugs because real life seems so mundane. Many professionals also fall into the same trap, often boosting for work not necessarily for play.

If you boost your chemistry unnaturally, your body's ability to boost itself diminishes almost every time you use the drug, regardless of the drug you choose. Although for a while the feeling is great, over time the boosting takes its toll — better to save your money and get high on life naturally.

nicotine

Nicotine is a strong brain-altering drug and ignoring the harmful health effects of smoking, such as heart disease and cancer, jeopardizes your chance of being a peak performer.

It's also no coincidence that the behavior of someone quitting smoking parallels those of someone with low serotonin including restlessness, fidgeting, poor concentration, preoccupation with food, putting on weight and insomnia. Nicotine takes over the work of serotonin whenever you're stressed — so increasing your serotonin levels when trying to quit will help.

alcohol

Alcohol is both a food and a drug so has good and bad effects. Most of the good effects are gained through moderate drinking and most of the bad are a result of excess. As a drug it acts on the central nervous system, which controls most of your actions, thoughts and emotions. Its numbing qualities were once used medically as an anesthetic, but in milder doses it creates a sense of well-being and relaxation. Alcohol is a depressant, not stimulant. If you drink too much you're likely to drop into the depths of despair. All your worst thoughts and negative emotions are amplified when you're drunk, which is why people often say that when someone is depressed and feeling miserable it's simply the alcohol talking.

Alcohol is made by the fermentation of fruits, vegetables and grains and in its purest form is a colorless liquid. It requires no digestion and is absorbed into the blood stream directly through the walls of your stomach and intestines. Alcohol is broken down in the liver at the rate of approximately 1/3 ounce per hour. The rest is released on the breath and in sweat and urine.

Surprising benefits of alcohol

One alcoholic drink a day relaxes the blood vessels and reduces the risk of heart disease. That wonderful "ahh" feeling you get at the end of a stressful day is a good indication that this is working for you. Red wine also contains elements that bathe your cells in antioxidants, rich anti-cancer agents. Alcohol itself isn't fattening. A "beer belly" is poorly named; it would be more appropriate to call it a "what-you-ate-when-you-were-drinking beer belly." Alcohol increases the levels of the enzyme lipo-protein lipase, which opens the fat cell. Alcohol doesn't get converted into fat (only fat goes into a fat cell) but fast tracks the storage of fat. Whenever the "in" door of the fat cell is open the "out" door is shut. So while alcohol itself isn't fattening, the presence of it in your blood prevents you losing fat.

Drinking too much alcohol will lead to alcohol dependency or alcoholism and can cause cirrhosis of the liver, a kind of scarring that decreases the efficiency of the liver. Alcohol has also been linked to certain cancers such as those of the stomach, esophagus and colon. Drinking too much can lead to brain damage and behavior changes resulting in accidents, suicide and violence. Drinking a small amount often is less harmful than frequent, or even occasional, binge drinking.

Excessive drinking also affects the kidney hormones, which control water loss, making you want to go to the bathroom more often when drinking. Alcohol irritates the lining of the stomach, which contributes to nausea and enlarges blood vessels in the brain, contributing to the hurt the next day. Some drinks, such as fortified wines, have chemicals such as histamines in them that may lead to headaches and nausea.

Spotting the danger signs

- Do you drink alone?
- Do you need a drink to perform a task or to cope with a particular person?
- Do you find it extremely hard to be in a social situation unless you have a few drinks?
- Do you rationalize about your drinking?
- Do you pretend to yourself that you drink less than you do?

If you answered "yes" to these questions you could have a drinking problem. You may need help from a professional treatment center or a self-help group such as Alcoholics Anonymous as it's important to overcome the psychological dependence as well as the physical addiction.

caffeine

I loved my coffee so much I think I overdosed on it. Over the years I upgraded to stronger and stronger blends. At first my panic or anxiety attacks seemed totally unrelated. It was only when I stopped drinking anything with caffeine in it that I noticed a major change. My partner and I were trying to start a family and had finally in frustration turned to IVF. She wanted to give her body every chance to become pregnant and I decided to join her in the diet initiatives. My anxiety levels dropped as I stopped drinking caffeine. Then when I started having caffeine again my anxiety levels began to creep up. Now I drink decaffeinated through the day and have one strong caffeinated coffee to start the day.

Like most people, you're probably a coffee drinker — if not, it's likely you drink tea or Coke or eat chocolate. Possibly you enjoy energy drinks like Red Bull, which contains 80 mg of caffeine per serving and packs the same punch as a strong cappuccino.

Although caffeine is addictive, most health experts agree that mild doses (less than 300 mg, or five cups, a day) of caffeine aren't a problem.

Spiking adrenaline

The feelings of adrenaline and the results of drinking a large cup of coffee are almost the same. You get a rush feeling, your temperature drops, you breathe faster, your liver dumps sugar into your system and you're off and running.

How much caffeine do you drink in a day?

Caffeine content per cup	
Tea	40-50 mg
Coffee	60-90 mg
Cola beverages	25 mg
Hot chocolate	25 mg
Adult energy drinks	50-100 mg

Whatever you drink, aim for less than 300 mg of caffeine a day

When you drink coffee, your brain goes into overdrive and your pituitary gland sends a message to the adrenal gland to send in adrenaline. If you're an adrenaline junkie you need to be careful how much coffee you drink — going overboard will fire off precious adrenaline that you may have been able to use later in a real emergency.

Caffeine headaches

When caffeine enters the brain, the brain's blood cells constrict, causing withdrawal headaches when you stop. This constriction can also, however, alleviate headaches that are vascular based such as tension headaches and migraines. For example, new mothers recovering from a particularly nasty epidural may be given a caffeine drip. If the needle of the epidural goes in a little too far it can nick the spinal cord causing a severe vascular headache.

how caffeine stops you sleeping

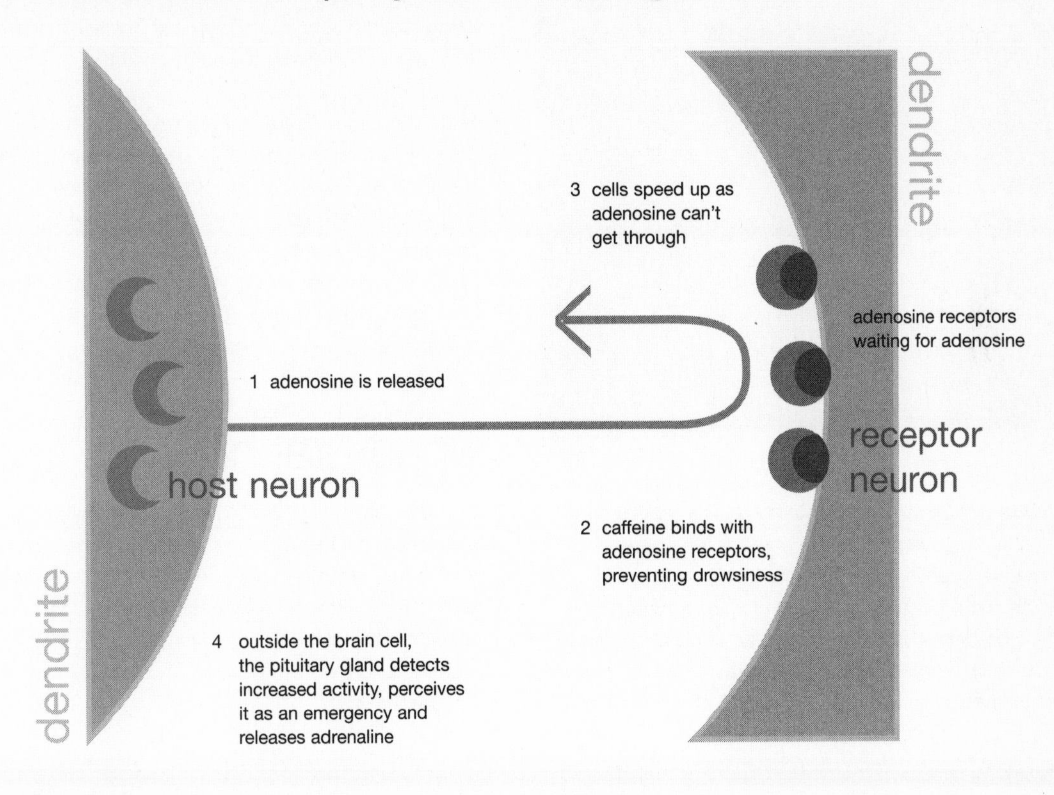

Going to the bathroom

Caffeine is a diuretic — it makes you urinate. So if you're trying to increase the amount of water in your diet, which is good for your health, caffeine is counterproductive. Not only does it cause your body to lose water, it will increase your trips to the bathroom during the day.

Depriving sleep

Caffeine actually resembles the brain chemical adenosine, which acts like a brain cell brake pad — one of its roles is to slow down brain cell activity, which in turn makes you drowsy. The brain has trouble telling the difference between adenosine and caffeine, even though there's actually a significant difference between the two.

big 5 replacements for unnatural highs

1. Drink green tea during the day for a lift without the caffeine hit.
2. Satisfy cravings by eating frequent, low-fat, high-protein mini-meals.
3. Eat fewer processed sugars and achieve a more even energy level.
4. To stay perky in the late afternoon, munch some licorice rather than dosing up on caffeine.
5. Instead of drinking booze to unwind late at night, try a cup of chamomile tea.

While adenosine slows down brain cell activity and makes you sleepy, caffeine parks in the adenosine reserved parking spots in your brain, stealing the coupling or receptor site held in place for adenosine. Having done this, it doesn't go on to do adenosine's job of slowing down brain cell activity. Rather, it keeps the car running all night. So instead of slowing down, your brain's cells go into overdrive. This is why coffee helps keep you awake. Although amphetamines are considerably more aggressive and obviously harmful, they work on basically the same process.

It takes about six hours for approximately half the caffeine you drink to be removed from your system. While some people can have a cup of coffee at night and still fall off to sleep, the depth of their sleep is in question. Caffeine hinders melatonin release from the pineal glands, disrupting the deep sleep that follows. Your sleep depth is what restores chemical imbalances throughout the day.

unnatural high

It's hard to make any kind of natural difference to your chemical profile if you seek unnatural highs. Illicit drugs, caffeine, nicotine and alcohol all affect your chemical balance — while the body can tolerate a certain level of caffeine and alcohol, nicotine and illicit drugs seriously mess with your body chemistry.

1 Drugs mess with your body's own natural chemicals and can prevent you from experiencing the wonderful natural process of feeling happy.

2 Nicotine mimics serotonin, which explains why quitters feel depressed, lack motivation, overeat and can't sleep at night.

3 Alcohol is a concentrated sugar and affects body chemistry dramatically. Have at least three alcohol free days a week.

4 Caffeine is addictive and stimulates adrenaline. It resembles the natural brain chemical adenosine, which slows down brain cell activity and prepares you for sleep — caffeine stops adenosine doing its job and stimulates you instead.

5 Caffeine constricts blood vessels and helps with vascular and tension headaches such as migraines, which explains why withdrawing from caffeine can lead to temporary headaches.

lights

Sleep is the best meditation.

DALAI LAMA

6

deep sleep

the power of sleep

Two of the most exciting things that could have happened to me both hit at once. I got the promotion to the marketing department and also became pregnant for the second time. I wasn't sure how the boss would take the pregnancy and I started to feel anxious about the "maternity leave conversation." This began to affect my sleep and I was afraid that with the morning sickness (which lasted all day) my boss would guess I was pregnant and take back the promotion. I wanted to tell her about being pregnant but it had to be when I was ready. I became more and more worried about how I was going to juggle a new job, a newborn, sleepless nights and a toddler. So I went back to basics and re-read my early child care books. One thing stood out loud and clear — the power of routine.

I started to have a bath at the end of the evening and adopt a newborn's pre-bed routine. Now I dim the lights and tone down the play with Nicholas. I got some up-to-date information about maternity leave and benefits. I'm now ready to have a conversation with my boss and negotiate a work plan for my return to work after the birth of our new baby. By adopting a routine and taking steps to fix my fear of talking to the boss I'm coping and sleeping so much better.

Sleep is one of the most important lifestyle factors for achieving great internal chemistry and a natural high. Deep sleep means you'll have greater productivity, better focus and more creativity. You'll be able to communicate ideas easily, have more energy and be willing to take on new tasks with less fear, staying happier throughout the day and remaining rational in crisis.

If you don't get enough sleep you become ill. Lack of sleep also causes horrific accidents, errors in judgment and is a major symptom and cause of depression. One night's missed sleep messes with your body chemistry for about six weeks as it can take that long for the body to return to a normal internal chemical balance and one hour lost every night for a week is the equivalent of staying up all night.

The sleep of success

Thomas Edison slept only a few hours each night and is still recognized as one of the most prolific inventors of our time. Einstein, on the other hand, said that he could not be creative on less than eleven hours sleep. Churchill used to squeeze in an hour-long midday power nap even during the war. Each of these highly successful men would have known his optimal amount of sleep and took responsibility for protecting the integrity of that sleep plan regardless of convention.

enough sleep

Each individual needs different amounts of sleep with the average adult requiring between three and ten hours. The amount of sleep you need also varies from week to week, depending on a variety of factors including how much sun you were exposed to during the day, the amount of exercise you did, and the degree of learning or new experiences you faced during the day. Although you may easily recognize the obvious sleep debt caused by working through the night, you may not be aware of the insidious creep caused by daily inadequate amounts of sleep. Finding out your optimal amount of sleep is a crucial step toward performing at your peak.

the science of sleep

When you're awake serotonin levels are at their peak. Then, as you pass into dream sleep, serotonin production stops. During the night the brain breaks down serotonin to create the powerful brain chemical melatonin. Serotonin acts like an accelerator during the day, keeping you happy and energetic, controlling when and what you eat. Melatonin acts like a parking brake during the night, allowing you to recuperate and letting your internal systems replenish themselves.

Melatonin is produced in the pineal gland by metabolizing serotonin. Its production is triggered by darkness and turned off by light striking the eye.

Mild sleep loss

You can't remember important details
You find it hard to pay attention
You lack energy

Moderate sleep loss

You struggle to string simple sentences together
You become irritated by little things
You can't regulate your temperature very well

Major sleep loss

You hallucinate
You fall asleep driving
You catch colds as your immune system plummets

SNAPSHOT

Melatonin is the key to deep sleep.

An adrenaline rush will make you tired and sleepy.

Too much serotonin in your system at night leads to restless sleep.

High levels of cortisol lead to disturbed nights and delayed bedtime.

After a big meal insulin kicks in and you're likely to feel sleepy.

are you getting enough sleep?

1 Do you fall asleep immediately when you go to bed or does it take 20 minutes or so to drop off?

2 Do you need an alarm clock to get up in the morning?

3 If you lie down for a nap in the middle of the day would you be asleep in less than 10 minutes?

4 Do your sleep patterns change on the weekends?

5 Do you find yourself sleeping for lengthy periods while on holiday?

Quiz key

1 If you drop off the minute your head hits the pillow, you could be forgiven for thinking that you're a good sleeper. But if you're getting an optimal amount of sleep each night, it should take you about 20 minutes to drop off.

2 To wake naturally before your alarm clock goes off is ideal and a good indicator that you're getting enough sleep. If occasionally during the week the alarm does wake you, your amount of sleep hasn't met your needs — using the alarm is a good security measure for this.

3 The middle of the day nap principle is simply a daytime equivalent of Question 1. If your answer to question 3 is "yes," you can safely say you're not getting enough deep sleep.

4 Often when we are getting insufficient sleep through the week, we sleep in at the weekend. This tends to simply shift the start of the day until an hour or two later. As a result, it's tougher to get going on Mondays.

5 Because of the stress throughout your normal day, you find that you want to catch up with lots of sleep when away from those stressors. While this is OK, it does indicate underlying problems with sleep debt in your "normal" life.

In animals, and presumably in humans as well, the production of melatonin can start or stop almost as immediately as the flick of a light switch. At night you have ten times the amount of melatonin circulating in your body as during the day. For all this to happen you need to be sleeping well.

Serotonin is necessary for voluntary muscle contraction, which is why your body stops circulating it during the night. People who sleepwalk have been shown to have active serotonin metabolites in their urine and blood after an episode. If serotonin were not switched off during the night you would begin to play out your dreams. One theory for dreams is that you're working through subconscious thoughts and sorting out a way of understanding them, replaying scenarios and adjusting your perceptions.

Daily activity and exercise cause wear and tear on your muscles and it's also during the sleep phase that your muscle tissue rebuilds and strengthens, so that the next time you overload them they'll be able to withstand the tension.

sleep waves

A typical night's sleep consists of the repetition of a one and a half to two hour cycle. A large part of this cycle is spent in non-dream sleep. Because metabolism and vital functions slow down during non-dream sleep, it's often called orthodox sleep. In contrast, REM or dream sleep, heightens brain activity.

During the two hour sleep cycle, you will progress through four key brain waves.

Beta waves

These are short sharp brain waves when you're awake and thinking. Most of your conscious time is spent in this state. Then, as you sleep more into the night, you should have fewer fully awake periods.

Alpha waves

When you meditate the brain is in an alpha state (although you don't have to be a meditator to experience this). If you've ever suddenly remembered something just as you began to fall asleep it's because your mind is relaxed — you're also more creative at this time.

Theta waves

Characterized by rapid eye movement (REM), this is dream sleep. In the late 1950s a physiological indicator of the dream state was found: at roughly 90 minute intervals, the eyes of sleepers were observed to move rapidly, and, at the same time, the sleepers' brain waves would show a pattern resembling the waking state. REM periods increase in length as the night progresses. REM sleep is thought to increase according to the amount of learning experienced during the day, possibly suggesting a memory function.

Delta waves

This is the deep sleep that's very restorative. You need to spend half of your sleep in this state (although in reality many people only get a quarter to one third of their sleep as delta sleep).

brain waves during sleep

beta
busy thinking,
conscious thought

alpha
relaxed, creative,
half asleep, half awake

theta
rapid eye movement,
dream state

delta
deep restorative sleep,
60 minutes is ideal

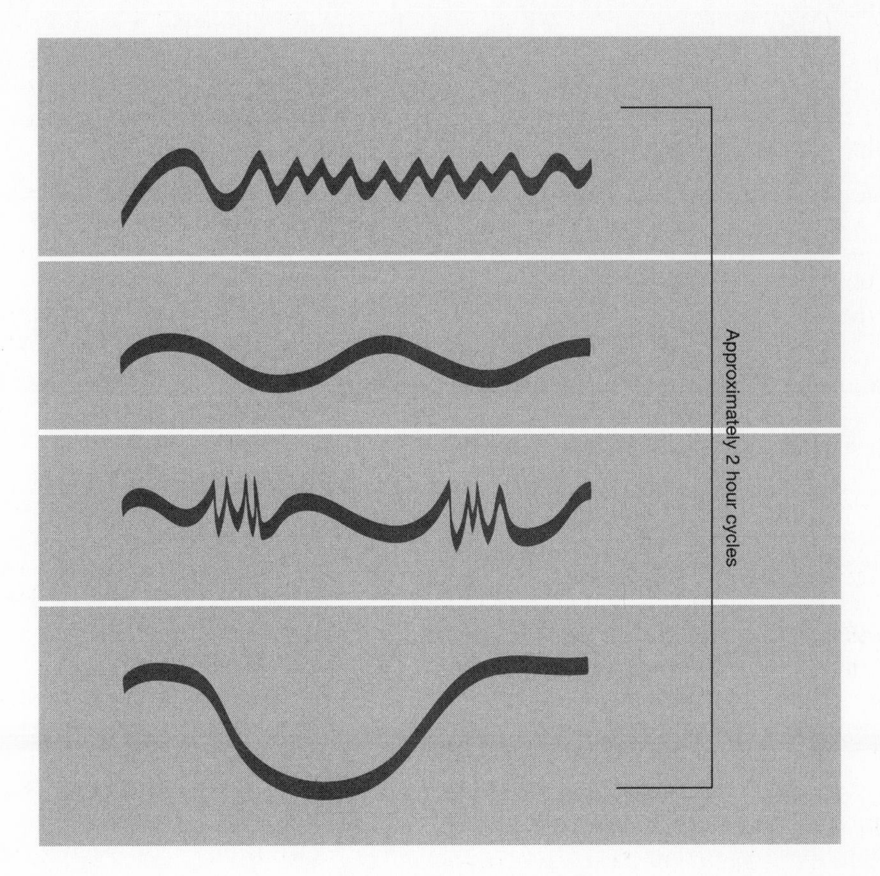

Aliens and demons

In an essay on alien abduction, Dr. Carl Sagan wrote that many people who claim to have been visited by aliens explain a waking paralysis "... as if the alien held me to the bed. I was awake but couldn't move a muscle." This paralysis is actually quite common. Your body has switched off serotonin in your muscles so that you don't act out your dreams. You feel paralyzed for a moment as your mind re-establishes the connection to your body. In medieval times there are accounts of demons sitting on the chests of sleeping victims. This is the same thing in a different era — they described demons while today's victims know demons don't exist so they see aliens from outer space.

insomnia

If you're unable to sleep enough to meet your needs you could be suffering from insomnia. If this is the case, it's particularly important you establish good sleeping habits. There are many causes of insomnia including stress, anxiety, depression and some psychiatric problems. Conditions such as asthma, heartburn, angina or other pain may also cause you to have trouble sleeping at night.

If you follow the general guidelines in this book for sleeping deeper, including creating a quiet, dark and comfortable sleeping environment; establishing a routine and exercising during the day; and practicing stress management, your insomnia should improve.

If you're suffering from insomnia, particularly if you're stressed, and wake up in the middle of the night, you might be tempted to do something like read the paper, fold laundry or watch TV thinking, "I'm awake so I might as well get something done." It's actually better to lie as quietly as possible and give your body a chance to learn to relax and hopefully resume the sleep cycle — especially if your adrenaline is pumping. If you're the type of person who thinks lying awake is wasting time, then you need the rest the most.

If you do get up you confuse your body's sleep–wake cycle. As you begin to move, your body starts the release of serotonin to help muscle contraction. Once serotonin starts to get active again, melatonin switches off and your chances of getting back to sleep are slim.

Jet lag

If you've traveled overseas and suffered jet lag you will have experienced the effect of lost sleep. As your body clock struggles to reset to the new time zone you feel sluggish and your head feels cloudy.

before you leave

Book your flight to arrive in the late afternoon or early evening whenever possible — if you're traveling east, aim to arrive early in the morning; if traveling west, aim to arrive later in the day. On your first night make sure you're in bed by 11:00 p.m.

on the flight

Drink plenty of water and minimize caffeine and alcohol during the flight. If you suffer from jet lag it may simply be you're dehydrated — the dry air of the plane, the caffeine and the booze all sap your body of water. Anticipate what time it is at the location you're traveling to. If it's night-time there then sleep on the plane, if it's daytime, stay awake.

when you arrive

Because temperature is the body clock's primary reset switch, keep the room a little cooler during the night and warmer in the morning.

Get outside in the morning, do some exercise and eat lightly regardless of how hungry you are.

Snoring

🔊 *My husband and I are compatible in most areas of our life together — except for our sleeping arrangements. I need my sleep environment to be perfect: quiet, dark and the temperature just so. Mike, on the other hand can nap anywhere, anytime. He can also snore! Unbelievably loud and long! Just as I'm dropping off into a beautiful relaxed sleep Mike starts. I nudge him to roll over and for a short time all is quiet. Then it starts again. I find myself listening, waiting for each intake of breath and the accompanying rattle and then virtually holding my breath for Mike to exhale. Most mornings I wake up exhausted.*

If you're in a deep restorative delta sleep you'll be enhancing your serotonin system so you can wake up happy and motivated. But if your partner snores and rolls over frumping the mattress and stealing the quilt, whether you're conscious of it or not, they have bumped you out of a deep delta sleep and interrupted your sleep cycle.

Consult a doctor and look into possible cures or devices to prevent snoring. More often than not, if you snore you need to exercise and lose weight.

sleeping deeper

Regardless of whether you're experiencing specific sleep problems, you can improve the quality of your sleep. Sleep is the number one way to restore your body balance — with great sleep you're assured a natural high.

Get in a rut about your sleep

The most important aspect of establishing a sleep routine is getting up at the same time every day and, if possible, waking into some daylight. Going to bed at the same time is less crucial, but certainly helps. If you're using "power naps," these should also be of a regular time and length. This lets your body establish a rhythm with its chemicals, so that you have plenty of adrenaline and serotonin available at the right times.

Ideally, maintain your sleep routine on weekends. The more regular you are, the better you will cope with the occasional disruption. Of course, if you travel, you should re-establish your routine as soon as you get home.

If you feel you may be in sleep debt, try adding hours to the start of your sleep cycle rather than the end and add your extra sleep in half-hour increments — go to bed half an hour earlier and see how your response is in the morning.

Relax before going to bed

Read a book, listen to soothing music or have a warm bath before you go to bed and only use your bed for sleeping. Avoid stimulants including tobacco, alcohol, tea, coffee or chocolate for at least four hours before sleep.

Avoid sleeping in

If you wake on some mornings later than normal you may actually wake feeling worse than if you had got up at your regular time. This could be because you've begun a new sleep cycle and haven't fully completed it. So, rather than rising into consciousness from a natural state of awakening, you force yourself out of deep sleep and into your day.

Or it could be that you're a busy person whose body is playing catch-up. Recognizing the extra rest, your body begins to come down off the adrenaline high and attempts to re-balance your chemical levels. With this re-balancing incomplete, you lack the drive of adrenaline to mask your exhaustion, and still lack serotonin levels as they have not had enough time to build up again. The groggy feeling could also be a combination of interrupting a sleep cycle and coming off the adrenaline high.

Make your bedroom dark

When it gets dark your brain begins to release melatonin so you sleep deeply. If you want better sleep you need to shut out light — the darker you can make the bedroom the better, as daylight sends a trigger to your brain to switch of melatonin production and begin manufacturing serotonin.

Artificial lighting, while generally not bright enough to turn on serotonin, is bright enough to prevent melatonin production.

Night masks may help, although if it's a hot night a sweaty face is a negative for your sleep environment. If you live in the center of the city, or are traveling and staying in a hotel, do what you can to block outside lights — a towel rolled up and placed at the bottom of the door will shut out light from hallways. Turn digital clocks with bright lights down or even turn them away from your line of sight.

When you're home, use candles for lighting and put dimmer switches on the lights — as the evening progresses turn down the lights. Read with a mini book light rather than a bright bedside lamp.

Control noise

Although controlling noise is a key element of the sleep environment, silence isn't always your goal. You'll quickly adapt to routine noise and are easily affected by a change in the routine — if you were to move to a house by the edge of a main road you would readily adapt to the hum of traffic while guests who visit for a couple of days would find it unbearable. If you live in the city and head to the country for the weekend the silence might be deafening.

Overhead ceiling fans and air-conditioning may all help dampen random noise. High quality earplugs also help level out noises that disrupt sleep, although they often take a little getting used to.

Regulate your body temperature in bed

Try to maintain a consistent body temperature when you sleep. Shake out your bed covering before you lie down to sleep so that the down and feathers are evenly distributed and have different summer and winter bed covers if your seasonal temperatures vary greatly. Wear nightwear made from natural fibers that breathe, such as cotton.

Your depth of sleep will be affected significantly if your partner has a different body temperature from yours. So cuddle your partner then dispatch them to their side of the bed. Consider separate bed covers if you and your partner are typically different temperatures when in bed.

Consider separate beds

If you both weigh more than 130 lbs. try sleeping on a king size bed or, better still, two single beds pushed together. Many couples, as they get older, sleep in separate beds as the need for quality sleep becomes crucial. As you age, the pineal gland makes less melatonin and you sleep less. Experts agree that physical exercise and maintaining muscle tissue can alleviate this decline and help you sleep better as you get older.

Eliminate bugs

Put your mattress out in the direct sunlight, as our ancestors used to do regularly, to debug it. Or you can have it debugged with a high voltage vacuum cleaner with a HEPA filter. People with asthma do this as a matter of course at least once a year, but everyone could achieve better quality sleep by doing this. Also refill or change your pillows often.

Make yourself at home when you travel

I work as a travel consultant, forever in and out of new and different accommodations. I became obsessed with the pillows in the various hotels I stayed in. The first thing I would check when I walked into yet another hotel room was the type of pillow on the bed. Some were hard and unrelenting, others too soft and yielding — the "just right" pillow was very elusive. After many a long disturbed night trying to bash a strange pillow into submission, I decided it was better to sacrifice some of my clothing requirements in my suitcase, and in their place pack my trusted favorite pillow. The result — every night seemed just as if I was happily tucked in my own bed — well, almost!

Sorting out your sleep environment means making it comfortable for you. It's well worth finding a pillow you like, taking it with you when you travel, along with photos and other bedside items, which connect you to your home environment.

Exercise during the day

Research has shown that you will sleep better at night if you exercise during the day, particularly aerobic exercise. If you don't sleep well at night, think seriously about making a brisk walk or light jog a part of your lunchtime plan. Exercise is a classic example of investing time in an activity to reap the rewards later — a one-hour workout makes your other 23 hours so much more effective.

the power nap

The siesta is a wonderful idea. For example, children in Spain go to school between 7:00 a.m. and 1:00 p.m. — this makes good sense as this is the peak mental time of the day. Body temperature begins to drop at 12:00 noon and stays down until about 3:00 p.m. The Spanish stop work during this time, go home, see the kids, eat a good meal, have a snooze and then attack the rest of the day with renewed vigor.

There can be enormous benefit from splitting your day like this. Similar to meditation, napping allows you to relax your mind. It gives your mind and body a chance to catch up with the demands put upon them during the day. If your work doesn't allow a power nap because of open plan offices or rigid 9 to 5 policies, you can still change focus in the middle of the day by taking a brief walk in the park or sitting on a bench outside for 20 minutes — it's a compromise to a nap but helpful anyway.

Experiment with ideal times of day and length of rest as this will vary from person to person. Be sure not to slip into a full-blown sleep cycle but rather doze for 30 to 45 minutes — interrupting a deep sleep cycle can cause you to wake feeling groggy and much worse than before.

If you're trying to overcome insomnia, it's better not to nap during the day as this is thought to shorten your sleep cycle in the evening, and if you're recovering from jet lag, make sure you return to your normal sleep patterns as soon as possible, even if you feel tired at the wrong times.

extra help for deep sleep

If you still find it difficult to sleep after trying all the strategies here, it's possible to supplement your melatonin but they are best used in bouts rather than a daily tonic like multivitamins.

Although melatonin supplements appear to help with better sleep it's not necessarily longer sleep. A recent study demonstrated that the differences between 0.01 mg and 10 mg dosages were not significant. In comparison, the average adult human produces 1 mg of melatonin in a 24-hour period whereas most tablets available through a pharmacist or health food store come in 3 mg dosages. Still a controversial subject, most experts agree regular use is a concern, although the side effects are not yet known.

Deep sleep

While Thomas Edison thought sleep was unnecessary, we now know it serves a vital function, restoring chemical balance and increasing vitality. Sleep is the ultimate downtime. Getting outside during the day, exercising regularly, minimizing stimulants like caffeine, and establishing a routine sleep–wake cycle will promote deep sleep. Focus on productive sleep hours and your awake hours will almost look after themselves.

lights

1 Getting enough regular sleep is crucial for achieving a naturally high life and maintaining good health.

2 A night's sleep is the repetition of a sleep cycle that lasts for about one and a half to two hours. Interrupting a cycle can have negative consequences.

3 Deep sleep repairs and regenerates functions to prepare you for the next day's activities.

4 A good indicator that you're getting enough sleep is a gradual falling to sleep over a 20 minute period and waking without an alarm clock.

5 When you sleep, melatonin, which is made from serotonin, is released from the pineal gland. When you're awake, serotonin aids in many functions including muscle contractions. Restless legs and fidgeting at night are often a result of a confused sleep–wake system.

Part of the secret of success in life is to eat what you like and let the food fight it out inside.

MARK TWAIN

7

mood foods

food and your current chemical balance profile

I have always treated food with a certain contempt — I just don't get excited by it. At the end of the day a frozen meal tossed in the microwave was about all I could do. If I got home after 8:00 p.m. I was more likely to have a bowl of breakfast cereal. I'm definitely an adrenaline junkie, wolfing down the food and trying to shut down the hunger. Then not long ago my partner had a health scare. To be supportive I decided to eat more organic unprocessed foods. I knew though that we had to work things into our hectic lifestyle so I started preparing soups, or at least buying fresh ones from our local deli, and this became a dinner. I also started to chop meal-size salads, chockfull of raw vegetables like carrot and cucumber. Then I would dump ham or turkey meat onto the top of the salad and sprinkle some nuts on as well. I have to admit I feel great — not only is my skin looking better but I'm waking up with so much more focus and vigor. I guess I just never realized how badly I was eating. I still don't get off on food but I'm feeling better than I have for years.

Each time you eat your body chemistry will be affected — you'll either get a high or a low depending on what you eat. Organic natural foods and eating frequently, will supply your body with the building blocks for great chemistry. If you simply eat what you know to be healthy, and cut out the fast foods, you'll have better energy levels, increased focus and will be able to shed excess weight. Although you don't need to know about mood foods to improve your general health, you can also use foods to help deal with depression, outsmart your fat cell and stem the strikes of hunger that often signal a chemical imbalance.

SNAPSHOT

When running on adrenaline you don't want to eat.

High levels of serotonin promote the feeling of being full or satisfied.

Cortisol increases your cravings for sweet and fatty foods.

Along with light and temperature when and what you eat sets your body clock so you know whether it's day or night – melatonin underpins this process.

Insulin protects the brain from excess sugar and also controls whether you store or lose fat.

the way you eat

The way you eat, not just what you eat, says a lot about your current chemical balance profile. If you're not hungry in the morning you're leaning toward adrenaline junkie, while if you have cravings for sugar, particularly in the afternoon, you're probably a serotonin seeker.

craving food — serotonin satisfaction

I knew it was going to be one of those days. I had four slices of toast with peanut butter and honey for breakfast but I still felt "down." The mall beckoned so I decided some serious retail therapy was the order of the day — the accounts could wait. I shopped frantically, knowing deep down that most of the things I bought were completely useless and would sit in a closet gathering dust. The simple cup of green tea I should have had became a creamy cappuccino, accompanied by rich carrot cake and lashings of whipped cream. Later that day it was munching on a big bag of jelly babies and indulging in serious window-shopping. Then I took off to the movies and ate a large popcorn and an ice cream. What a day! Sometimes I can't seem to focus on what I need to do and then I just pig out — nothing I eat or do seems to satisfy me. I still have these uncontrollable cravings on certain days but now I try to have emergency fiber foods, like my apricots, in case I get a craving. Often I still have a sweet snack after the apricots but I don't binge to the same degree. I've also started eating more protein — the days I forget to do this are the worst!

Which of the following four eating patterns resembles the way you eat?

A I eat three meals a day and rarely between meals or after the evening meal.

B I eat three meals a day and one or more between meals or after meal snacks.

C I don't start eating until late afternoon and dinner, then eat until I go to sleep.

D I nibble all day and rarely eat meals.

Answers

A = Balanced profile
B = Serotonin
C = Adrenaline/cortisol profile
D = Cortisol/serotonin profile

Serotonin (along with several other chemicals) triggers the brain when you're full or satisfied, so if you're low in serotonin you may crave food. This means that hunger can be a poor indication of when you need to eat because your regular eating patterns, and moods, often determine your hunger rather than any physiological need for food. If your body is hungry, it will tell you to eat whatever is available — chocolate cake or a bowl of broccoli.

If you have a serotonin personal profile you'll often have a craving mid-afternoon for sugars. The brain is trying hard to get tryptophan so it can manufacture your happy chemical serotonin. But if you have too

the great day diet

6:30 a.m. A glass of water to start the day.

You need at least 8 glasses of water during the day so get your count going early.

7:00 a.m. Breakfast of fruit and/or low glycemic index, slowly digested cereals such as bran flakes or shredded wheat and skim milk.

Twice a week have a low fat high protein breakfast. Omelettes are a great way to achieve this.

9:00 a.m. Another glass of water.

9:30 a.m. 1 to 2 cups of coffee. A teaspoon of sugar is fine — 2 to 4 per cup is overdoing it. Chase every coffee with a glass of water.

If you're an adrenaline junkie, limit the amount of caffeine you have in the mornings. If you have a melatonin profile, consider avoiding caffeine altogether.

10:30 a.m. Crackers with tomato and cheese, or tinned tuna or salmon. Maybe a blend of egg white, skim milk powder and a fruit of your choice.

12:30 p.m. High protein, low carbohydrate lunch of salad and fish or turkey. A glass of water.

1:30 p.m. Another glass of water.

2:30 p.m. Bowl of oatmeal with a little honey on it or 2 fruit bread rolls (no butter).

4:30 p.m. Another glass of water and a piece of fruit (watermelon is perfect).

6:30 p.m. Bowl of nuts and a glass of wine or a beer (choose almonds and walnuts).

7:00 p.m. A dinner of a large minestrone soup and a sourdough bread roll, or lean meat and bowl of steamed vegetables. A glass of water.

9:00 p.m. Slice of toast with jam or honey and a cup of decaffeinated tea.

10:00 p.m. Peppermint or camomile tea.

ALL DAY snack on a trail mix combination of roasted oats, seeds, nuts and dried fruit. A bag of dried fruit like apricots also helps balance cravings and a bag of snow peas or green beans raw will help stem hunger.

Good snacks for breaking hunger
a bowl of All-Bran or rough breakfast cereal
a low sugar muesli bar
an apple
rough, heavy, unprocessed bread with big grains
hard-to-chew vegetables like broccoli and cauliflower

much sugar, or mix the sugar with a fat in the form of a chocolate bar, you disable the serotonin hit.

It's especially frustrating when you're trying to lose weight but feel hungry all the time — you may be tempted to skip breakfast to put off the "hunger pains" because when you eat frequently you'll tend to feel hungry more often. But constant hunger shows that your metabolism is firing, which is a good thing. Your body is like a furnace — you stoke the fire, making it hotter every time you put something in your mouth.

The key to controlling hunger is to respond with low-fat, high-fiber foods. Don't respond by putting in fat and quickly digested sugars as they're an inefficient fuel that increases the fire but creates waste the body has to dispose of. While this fuel may increase your metabolism, you also end up with more unnecessary fat to eliminate. You can eat sweets, desserts and junk food as a conscious treat — when you're in control, not when you're hungry.

making serotonin

Making more serotonin in your brain is a four-step process. How you organize your lifestyle can influence the first two steps — steps 3 and 4 simply happen after that.

Step 1 You eat food rich in the amino acid tryptophan such as turkey, almonds and red meat, to ensure tryptophan is present at the blood brain barrier.

Step 2 Insulin clears excess fat, sugar and proteins from the area so that tryptophan can cross over to the brain unimpeded.

Step 3 The tryptophan is converted into a smaller substance called 5-htp and crosses over.

Step 4 In the brain, 5-htp is transformed into serotonin by another chemical.

You can help your brain make serotonin by eating 300 mg to 600 mg a day of tryptophan-rich food and having a sugar hit. Although sugar or carbohydrates are necessary to trigger the release of insulin, be careful you don't overdose on quickly digested sugars as this will leave you tired and lethargic (low blood sugar) rather than giving you a serotonin high.

So for a natural high, review your diet to see if you're getting enough tryptophan and have a controlled sugar hit in the afternoon.

Eat tryptophan-rich food

The brain creates most neurotransmitters from amino acids (found in protein-rich foods), which are the building blocks for cell construction. Your body needs eight "essential" amino acids from which to create the other "non-essential" amino acids. Animal proteins contain all eight essential amino acids whereas vegetable proteins (such as nuts, peas or dried beans) do not. If you're a vegetarian you need to make sure you get enough essential amino acids by eating a mixture of protein sources.

Two major amino acids that create many neurotransmitters are tyrosine and tryptophan. Tyrosine makes the excitory brain chemicals dopamine and adrenaline, which act on brain cells to get you going. Tryptophan makes the calming or inhibitory chemicals, melatonin and tryptamine.

Once eaten, the food needs to travel through the intestinal system into the blood stream and make its way to the brain where it then has to cross over.

Have a sugar hit

To enable tryptophan to cross over to the brain you need a pure hit of about 40 g of quickly digested sugar. Your body signals this process by craving for sugar — these sugar cravings, which usually occur mid-afternoon, are a result of your brain's desire to make more serotonin. The sugar creates a controlled release of insulin into the blood stream, the insulin rushes through your system clearing out sugar then stores it in your liver and muscles in the form of glucose and glycogen. At the same time it causes fatty acids to move into the fat cells for storage and deals with other protein molecules in your blood that are not able to cross the blood brain barrier. Once the blood near the brain barrier is clear of other amino acids, tryptophan and tyrosine are able to cross over.

Foods rich in tryptophan

Protein	Serve	Mcgs of tryptophan
Almonds	100 g	170
Cheddar cheese	250 g	330
Chicken	100 g	390
Cottage cheese	250 g	300
Ground beef	100 g	320
Kidney beans	250 g	180
Lentils	250 g	160
Milk	200 ml	110
Pork	100 g	390
Salmon	100 g	250
Scrambled eggs	2 eggs	200
Soy milk	200 ml	110
Soy protein powder	2 tablespoons	220
Tempeh	100 g	310
Tofu	100 g	280
Tuna	100 g	320
Whole-wheat spaghetti cooked	500 g	190
Yogurt	200 ml	70

not hungry — adrenaline junkies

I don't know how it happened but I woke up one day and I was over 225 pounds! Now I know it didn't happen overnight but it did creep up on me. Work had been full on and we had just finished renovating the house. But things were going well — I had started to see money in the bank and was happy with my relationship. I used to eat 3 to 4 meals a day religiously but in the last year or so I had begun to skip lunch and eat on the run later in the day, living off coffee and "unwinding" with drinks after work. What still amazes me to this day is how I could put on weight when I didn't eat regular meals. After seeing a nutritionist and filling out a week's food diary I got a rude shock. Because I was on the go so much I was choosing high fat food full of processed sugars that quickly satisfied the need to eat. Even though I ate less often I was eating calorie dense food and so piled on the weight. I now take time to eat, and eat well, before I pig out. A simple thing but it helped me drop down to 205 pounds — at least a move in the right direction.

If you're on the adrenaline side of the current chemical balance profile you'll usually wake instantly alert, a to-do list rolling through your mind as you take a shower and get ready for the day. This instant "on" turns off appetite control and your body, using the stress response, supports the mental desire to hit the ground running. It holds off hunger and creates space for the fight. But if you skip breakfast the stress response you create in your body depletes much needed reserves of adrenaline and you might find you're not hungry until say 1:00 p.m.; whereas if you have breakfast at 7:00 a.m. you'll be hungry again at 11:00 a.m.

High performance sugar hits

1 cup of cooked vermicelli
3 slices of white bread
1 medium potato
4 large shredded wheat
1 Clif bar or 1 Clif shot
1/3 cup of raisins
2 large bananas
13 dried figs

Each of the high performance sugar hits is equivalent to a 40 to 50 g carbohydrate dosage. 40 g of a low fat carbohydrate is likely to cause the controlled sugar hit that allows insulin to clear out the blood stream and allow for the crossover to occur. Choose one from the list, stick to the quantities recommended and only use in the afternoons — there's not much point in hitting your body first thing in the day or at night. Limiting these foods after sunset will also help control your weight and energy.

the fat instinct

Humans appear to have a survival instinct to eat fat. Galanin, a neuropeptide that causes you to eat or crave fat, is released when you eat fat or go without eating for a period of time. This explains why, when eating a packet of chocolate cookies, there's a tendency to eat the whole packet rather than stop at just one — each fatty cookie builds the galanin crave for the next one.

Fat is OK — you need some fat on your body and in your diet to function. Without a certain amount of fat you also wouldn't be able to transport vitamins A,D,E and K (essential to vision, skin condition, getting energy from the food you eat, bone density and blood clotting) around your system. These four key vitamins are fat soluble, which means they're absorbed with the help of fats and stored in fat.

But if you're carrying excess weight you'll feel low because you're placing extra load on all your physical systems. Losing unwanted fat is a crucial step in achieving and maintaining a natural high but the worst message you can send an overweight body is to cut out fat by simply not eating. A lack of good nutrition, and infrequent eating, sends a message to your body instructing it to store fat and go into survival mode. This pushes up cortisol levels and depletes adrenaline levels.

If you're stressed, or running on cortisol, you'll crave fatty food, mainly due to the effect elevated cortisol has on appetite. Strong links between stress and obesity have also been identified — men who suffer prolonged stress are prone to fatty deposits around the midsection.

the fat cell

The fat cell is a room with a front door "in" and a back door "out." The "in" door of the fat cell is regulated by the enzyme lipoprotein lipase (LPL). By identifying the presence of this fat-storing enzyme, scientists have been able to examine what we eat and do to store fat. The partner enzyme to LPL is hormone sensitive lipase (HSL), which opens the fat cell to release stored fats into the blood stream to use as energy.

Storing fat

All fats you eat have the potential to be stored in a fat cell — some are held captive while others (such as avocados and olive oil) are more readily released into your system for use as energy. Fat in animal products creates free fatty acids which lead to high cholesterol and increase the risk of high blood pressure and heart disease. Your body tries to get these fats out of your blood and store them in the relative safety of the fat cell.

When you put sugar in your body, insulin is released. Once insulin is released everything else in your system, including fat, clears out of the way to make room for this brain-saving exercise. Your fat cells suck in the drifting fat in your blood, allowing the insulin to sweep through, attacking the blood sugars unimpeded (the same thing happens when you drink alcohol).

When you fail to eat, the fat cell flies into fat-storing mode. Nutritionists agree that this occurs when you eat less than 1200 to 1500 calories in a day. When deprived of food, your body begins a starvation response. Believing that you're about to head into a prolonged famine, it stores fat for survival by fast

outsmarting the fat cell

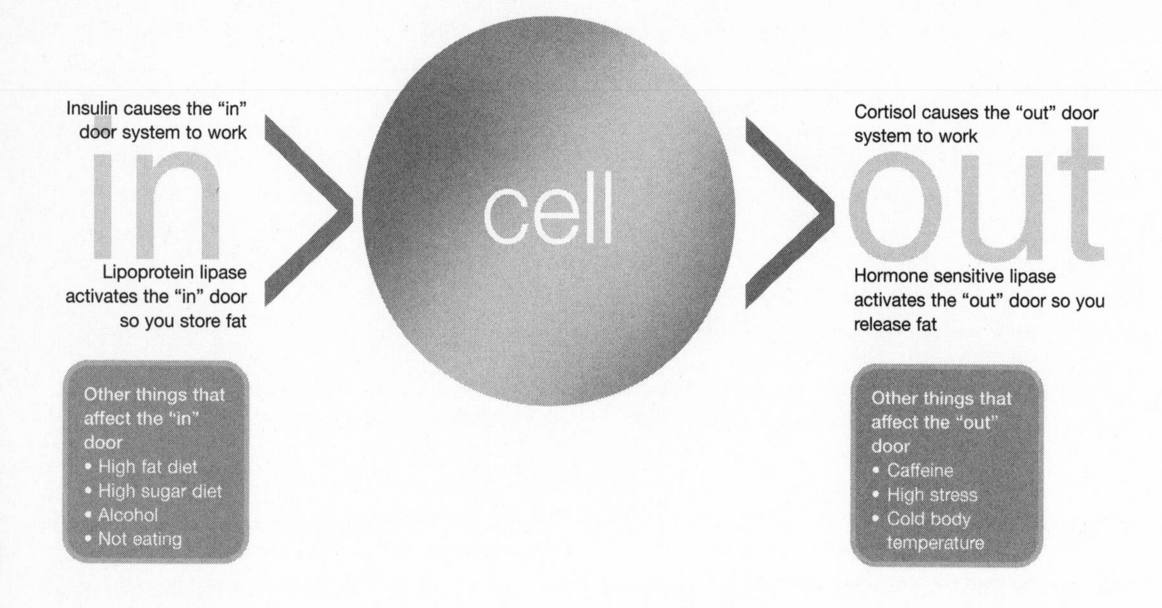

tracking any excess fat lying around in your blood-stream and digestive system to your fat cells.

Fat releasing

If you're physically fit you'll have higher levels of the fat-releasing enzyme HSL in your bloodstream as you demand more energy to stay alive. Your body prepares to meet these demands by making fat stored in the cells easily accessible at times of need. So it's easier to lose fat if you have a higher fitness level.

Fat is one of the best sources of energy in the body. Although improving your fitness will have a greater impact, when you're cold and stressed your body makes it easier for you to release fat and use it as fuel.

Caffeine also affects the use of fat as a fuel. Most commercial weight loss pills have varying amounts of caffeine in them. The average diet pill contains 250 mg of caffeine with the recommended dosage being approximately 2 to 4 tablets per day, causing

Can sugar and alcohol be converted into fat?

De-novo lipogenesis is the process of converting sugar into fat. While more research needs to be done in this area, there is evidence that it takes a lot of sugar before this occurs. Sugar and alcohol act as keys to unlock the fat cell so that the fat you eat is more readily stored.

your daily caffeine intake to exceed 1000 mg. This is far too high, even excluding the caffeine in the foods and beverages you would typically consume during a day. If you have less than 300 mg of caffeine per day your HSL levels rise and you can positively affect the release of fat from its stored form in the fat cell.

the GI rating

The Glycemic Index (GI), a rating of carbohydrates or sugars based on how quickly your body digests them, has changed the way we look at sugars and redefined eating for weight loss or energy gain.

Quickly digested sugars and carbohydrates are likely to push your blood sugar levels up dramatically and force the release of insulin. But if the carbohydrate is slow to be digested insulin release is prevented and you'll have a slow energy release throughout the day.

Particularly if you identified insulin and sugar sensitivity in your current chemical balance profile, you can use this information to regulate your blood sugar levels more closely.

Factors affecting the speed of sugar digestion

1. How rough and unprocessed the food is. Unprocessed rugged foods such as whole-grain breads are slower to digest than highly refined white breads.

2. How fatty the food is. Fat tends to slow down the rate of digestion. Foods with a low GI but high fat content (for example potato chips versus raw potato) are not necessarily the best foods for balancing your body chemistry.

3. How you cook the food. If you grind foods down or remove their skins and coatings (say washing down rice) you'll speed up the rate it can be broken down and the effect on your blood sugars.

4. How starchy the food is. Some starches are slower to break down than others and may affect how fast you digest the foods you eat.

Sample GI rating

Food	GI
Brown rice	66
White rice	72
Spaghetti	42
Fructose	30
Honey	87
White bread	69
Whole-wheat bread	72
Rye bread	42
Pastry	59
Apple	39
Bananas	62
Cherries	23
Grapes	45
Peaches	29
Raisins	64
Grapefruit	26
Oranges	40
Skim milk	32
Baked beans	40
Carrot	92
Lentils	29
Frozen peas	51
Potato chips	51
Potato	70
Mars Bar	68

50+ = foods that enter the blood stream more quickly. 50- = foods that enter the blood stream more slowly. These low GI sugars will give you more energy throughout your day.

the importance of vitamins and other supplements

If the three basic nutrients (fats, proteins and sugars) are the fuel for the body, then vitamins and minerals are the oils, lubricants and additives for peak performance. By themselves they do very little, but in conjunction with good eating and exercise they contribute significantly to balancing your body chemistry and general good health. For example, people often think that Vitamin B is the energy vitamin, but by itself B gives no energy. What it does is help extract energy from the foods you eat.

If you eat well and are consistent with your eating patterns you won't need vitamin and mineral supplements because you'll get all the vitamins and minerals you need straight from the food you eat. But if you miss meals and don't eat a variety of foods you may benefit from vitamin and mineral supplements.

Some people criticize vitamin supplements saying they're simply creating expensive urine because the vitamins rush quickly through the body and are passed out without being effective. Although it's true you do waste a lot of the vitamins you're paying for, you can slow this process by taking vitamins with food and using brands that attempt to reduce the speed of digestion.

Taking vitamin supplements is simply a blanket insurance policy to make sure you're giving your body an environment where it can choose to either accept or reject the vitamins it may need. For a busy modern lifestyle it's not too high a cost to ensure that you're operating at peak efficiency and insuring yourself against neglect. Some vitamins (such as C) can't be stored and so, unless you eat the right foods on a particular day, you'll definitely need a supplement. With other vitamins you may need to replenish reserves from time to time.

Some people believe that advocating vitamin supplements encourages the belief that healthy eating is not necessary, that it's OK to eat poorly — simply pop a pill and everything will be fine. While it's true that you only need vitamins if your dietary intake is inadequate, replacing vegetables with a pill is not an option because you miss much of the necessary fiber and you're getting a second-rate vitamin. Nothing beats vitamins the way nature intended us to have them, so you must eat well.

There's also no point having a bad day and then taking supplements. It's too late — your body needed the vitamins to perform functions during the high stress day. Better to be honest about the day ahead and accept that you're not going to eat well. On a day of deadlines and crisis management, popping a pill in the morning as a second rate vitamin intake may make a difference.

B vitamins and depression

When you run on adrenaline and cortisol your body is sapped of extra vitamins and minerals. Vitamin B complex, magnesium and zinc are needed for circulation and blood sugar control — if you don't maintain your levels of these the stress escalates. Depressed people have been shown to have B12, B2, B6 deficiencies. When you're depressed you don't feel much like eating, so it's not clear which comes first, the depression or the deficiency. But several studies have shown that supplementing with B complex vitamins, or having B12 shots, makes a difference to depression. Taking vitamin B supplements when you're depressed will help you achieve a natural high.

final mood food tricks

Protein rocks

If you eat fish three times a week, grill meats and eliminate oils, your staple proteins will become great helpers in the quest for a naturally high life without the need for going on a fad protein diet. Cutting back on processed carbohydrates and increasing lean proteins helps you think clearly, and control hunger and weight loss.

Smart fish

Known as omega oils (omega-3), the oils in fish make up more than half the fats found in the brain cell receptor sites for neurotransmitters. If you eat 100 grams of fish three times a week, your body receives its optimal amount of omega-3 and your brain chemistry has more places to dock and deliver its messages. You'll think more clearly, be more alert and generally happier if you eat fish.

Love affair with chocolate

True dark chocolate is low in sugar and high in mood food effect. Phenethylamine (which is found in all

Three ways to get your vitamins

Nature's way

Five to six times a day, eat a diet rich in a variety of fresh vegetables, lightly cooked. Munch on two or three pieces of fruit during the day and have vegetable crudités before dinner at night. Always shop for the freshest produce.

The investigator's way

Look at the vitamins contained in foods and consider what your typical diet is and where there is a deficiency. Then buy and consume only those vitamins that you lack.

The lazy way

If you find it all too hard and can't be bothered preparing fresh vegetables daily or examining what you eat, simply buy a good multivitamin and take it each morning. Do this weekdays and on the weekends but work on getting a natural intake of foods instead of taking multivitamins. Because your fiber intake is lower when you don't eat fresh vegetables, have a bowl of breakfast cereal that is high in bran and dietary fiber. The label will tell you how much fiber is in a serving — you need 30 g of dietary fiber a day. Nature's way is still the best option, but the lazy way is better than doing nothing.

chocolate) helps produce adrenaline via its precursor impact on dopamine and has also been shown to improve women's sexual function.

Stimulating licorice

Licorice is a natural stimulant that stops your body breaking down cortisol, keeping you on edge. This can be useful if you need to stay "on" and are not suffering from stress, but it's not good if you're a burnout candidate.

Siberian ginseng

All types of ginseng help people suffering from adrenal fatigue as it elevates your stress threshold. Because of its potency, only use it during high stress periods rather than all year round. Most naturopaths recommend Siberian ginseng over the Asian type, particularly for women.

mood foods

Once you've sorted out your sleep, focus on what you eat. Become aware of the chemical consequences of your diet — how you eat also points to a particular chemical balance profile. Skipping breakfast is a trait of the adrenaline junkie while craving sugar mid afternoon is typical of a serotonin seeker. You can change your mood through your food.

1 How you eat during the day is indicative of your current chemical balance profile. For example, if you skip breakfast you're probably an adrenaline junkie.

2 Adrenaline suppresses your hunger until you actually eat — high cortisol makes you choose fatty food.

3 The satisfied feeling you get after eating is often a result of elevated serotonin levels.

4 Some sugars are digested more slowly than others. These low GI sugars will give you even more energy throughout your day and an enduring natural high.

5 Through your diet you can influence the availability of proteins and insulin, two important steps in the making of serotonin.

6 The fat cell is opened to store fat by the enzyme LPL and opened to release fat by the enzyme HSL. This knowledge helps to outsmart the fat cell and balance body chemistry.

7 Carrying excess body weight decreases your chemistry for success — losing excess weight will help you feel naturally high.

Whenever I get the urge to exercise

I lie down and it goes away.

WINSTON CHURCHILL

8

Churchill's urge

a natural "rush"

🔊 *Lately I've become edgy and uptight by the end of the working day. Traveling home to see the kids I would think how much I love them, then the minute I walked through the door I'd yell at one of them. At the urging of a very close friend I started going to the gym a few days a week. This has now increased to every day. It has become the thing I do to unwind before I get home. The kids call the workouts "Dad's medicine" – they know that if I don't go for a run or miss a workout a few days in a row I'm going to be a grouch. My daughter even now helps me pack my gym bag in the mornings.*

You'll get so much more out of life if you exercise. Exercise creates a "rush" without the need for artificial stimulants. By doing regular and different types of exercise, you'll increase your levels of the happy chemical serotonin, improve your stress tolerance by burning off stress chemicals such as cortisol, and sleep deeper by manufacturing more melatonin. Regular exercise provides you with more energy, will make you stronger and fitter, and less prone to injury. It can improve mild to moderate depression as well as balance sugar responses (insulin) giving you even and consistent daily energy. There's also evidence that the cardiovascular benefits of exercise promote a longer life.

If you work in a high pressure job you're especially at risk if you don't exercise, as high levels of cortisol will make you uptight and edgy. And if cortisol levels rise unchecked they can lead to heart disease, cancer, diabetes, depression and other debilitating illnesses. Much compulsive behavior is also attributed to high cortisol and low serotonin levels.

Are we fit?

According to studies done in 2002 by the U.S. Department of Health and Human Services, 59% of American adults reported that they did not engage in any kind of vigorous, leisure-time physical activity. Based on their Body Mass Index (BMI), an estimate of total body fat calculated from height and weight, 35% of American adults were overweight and 23% were obese.

Common excuses given for not exercising: "no time," "fear of injury," "lack of motivation," "family obligations," "no experience," "can't afford," "no persistence," "no company," and "don't enjoy."

hissy fit

If you've ever had a slow leak in your car's tires, you'll notice that the air gradually hisses out of the tire and the car becomes more difficult to drive. The changes in the car's performance are small and they creep up on you — it's not until you actually put air back into the tires that you realize how bad things had become or how good things could be.

Frequent exercise has the same effect. Just like the air slowly hissing out of the tire, the benefits of exercise take some time to appear — and also take a while to disappear once you stop exercising. Although investing in regular exercise will mean higher quality of life — a natural high — don't expect it to happen as an immediate result of each exercise session. You won't notice significant changes until you've been exercising regularly for about six weeks.

Is your fitness creeping away?

1. Do you get out of breath when you walk up three flights of stairs?
2. Are you finding it harder to carry the groceries from the car to the kitchen?
3. Are you getting tired and stiff when you sit in a long meeting?
4. Do you still enjoy physical play with your kids or do you get tired in the first 10 minutes and have to stop?
5. Are you ready to sleep each night or do you become restless and fidgety?

If you answered "yes" to any of these, your youthful fitness may be slipping away. Fitness is often ignored as you get on with life and only becomes apparent when you stop to think about it.

Because the efforts and rewards of exercising aren't obviously linked, some people find it a struggle to "commit to get fit." Focusing on how you look will only stimulate you while you're young and gorgeous or going through a midlife crisis. Forget the aesthetics of exercise — life is too short to be looking in the mirror all the time! But exercising because you're afraid of a heart attack isn't good motivation either. So focus on the thought that exercising will make you feel and function so much better.

fighting the big excuses

I'm not motivated

If you find it hard to get started on exercise, put your exercise clothes on when you get up and don't take them off until you exercise. Or don't eat your lunch until you've done some exercise. Alternatively, sweep your front porch or mow the lawn and at work plan errands that require walking during your lunch hour.

I don't have time

Include movement by walking up stairs instead of taking the elevator, getting off the bus a few stops before home or walking to the shops instead of driving. If you take your children to sports, walk around the track or help with coaching.

If you're a morning person go for a swim or take a brisk walk before work. When you're at work, talk to people in person rather than use the telephone or email, and hand deliver messages. At lunchtime, workout with a friend — try swimming, aerobics, walking or jogging. Then in the evening, involve neighbors, family or friends in a walk around the block.

I'm not the sporty type

You don't need any special skills to exercise. For most people walking is the easiest exercise. If you don't want to play team sports or go to a gym, swimming, cycling, bowling and jogging are all activities you can do when you feel like it.

SNAPSHOT

Adrenaline is used in most competitive high energy exercise activities.

Serotonin levels can be increased with rhythmic low intensity activity.

Excess cortisol levels are lowered when you exercise.

Melatonin is manufactured when you exercise, so exercise helps you sleep better.

Exercise moderates the need for insulin dumps, so you stay more alert and focused.

I'm scared of injuring myself
If you exercise sensibly by warming up, cooling down and stretching, you can avoid injury. Start with easy exercises and build up gradually and don't exercise if you're ill. Also see a doctor if you want to exercise hard and you're a man over 35, or a woman over 45; exercise causes chest pain; moderate exercise makes you breathless; or if you have heart disease.

energy pathways

Your body gets the energy it needs from the food you eat by extracting energy from the fats, sugars and proteins in your diet. Because protein is a poor source of energy, fats and sugars are the two main energy sources. The body uses sugars whether you need a lot or a little energy; fats are mainly used in the easy everyday activities or long but comfortable exercise sessions.

While the energy itself comes from food, the energy systems can be made more effective through exercise. By exercising, in particular the kind of exercise that makes you fitter aerobically, you begin to handle with ease activities that previously left you breathless — your everyday activities are burning fat as a fuel.

The body stores energy in the form of adenosine triphosphate (ATP), sometimes called the basic currency of energy in the human body as all forms of energy are derived from this one tiny substance — your body will get energy in many different ways but in the end all it really wants is ATP.

ATP, or energy, is made through three basic pathways: the ATP-CP system and the aerobic and anaerobic systems. These three systems operate like a three-lane highway with a fast, medium and slow lane. Depending on your energy needs at the time, your body can switch systems from the slow (aerobic) to the medium (anaerobic) and fast (ATP-CP) system. Often you ride the lines between lanes using a combination of the systems.

The ATP-CP system

The ATP-CP system uses creatine phosphate and produces enough energy for about 30 seconds of activity. Creatine phosphate is like gunpowder sprinkled throughout your muscles — it gives off a flash of quick energy and then rapidly burns out. Many quacks and charlatans claim to have developed powders and tablets that boost creatine phosphate stores. Your body actually creates its own creatine phosphate from the food you eat — there are no magic solutions to add to it.

The aerobic and anaerobic systems

What you eat and do can have a dramatic effect on the aerobic and anaerobic systems. When you need energy for low intensity activity your body uses the aerobic system. Under this system your body uses sugars and fats as fuels to supply you with energy. A very efficient system — your body breaks down the fuels and leaves you with carbon dioxide (which you breathe out) and water (which you pass, use or store). You mainly use this system in everyday activities — it's a slower burner, ticking over at a low but constant level.

When your body needs energy in a hurry, but for longer than the 30 second period provided by the gunpowder-like creatine phosphate, it gets it through the anaerobic system. Using sugar as its fuel, this energy system is in such a hurry it doesn't completely break down the sugars it uses and leaves a waste product, lactic acid. Lactic acid is that burning feeling you get when you're doing tough exercise like riding up a long hill on a bike. It can make you feel nauseous and cause temporary pain. Ninety percent of the lactic acid produced by your body is removed within an hour and is not the cause of pain the next day — this is delayed onset muscular soreness.

If you've ever been walking at a steady comfortable pace, and then had to climb a hill, you will have felt the shift from the aerobic to the anaerobic system.

Runners' high

People have been claiming for years that regular exercisers achieve a euphoric calm during and after exercise — the famed runners' high. The theory is that the body releases "endorphins" during the exercise and that these make you feel "high." Endorphins do create a morphine effect, which eliminates much of the pain the runners would otherwise feel. But there have been no significant findings to suggest that the average recreational athlete would have elevated levels of endorphins in their system either after or during a workout. The only people who have shown slightly elevated levels of endorphins are long distance runners — the prolonged duration was the determining factor in the release of these natural painkillers.

The feel good that happens after exercise is a result of the impact exercise has on cortisol and serotonin levels. It removes cortisol therefore eliminating tension and increases serotonin, promoting calm and well-being.

The benefits of spontaneous activity

Park car 1 mile from office and walk to work (5 days)	940 cals
Climb stairs at work instead of elevator, 4 floors (5 days)	500 cals
Walk the dog 1 mile a day (7 days)	330 cals
Walk to the grocery store for milk and bread (2 days)	185 cals

The aerobic system has adjusted itself to the demands of the walk, but is unable to quickly adjust to the new load. The anaerobic system kicks in to make up the difference — the symptoms of increased breath rate and burning muscles let you know this is happening. If the hill continues for a while, the anaerobic system may not last the distance. In this case you're forced to slow down to a level that the aerobic system can handle.

get moving for high performance

My friend Josh works out at the local gym and was always encouraging me to go along. I eventually did go one day — but it wasn't for me. The body-hugging outfits, mirrors and dauntingly fit bodies actually demotivated me. I used this as an excuse for the next year not to exercise at all! I've also never been into sports and was always the last one picked on any sporting teams — but then I found swimming. The anonymity of swimming with goggles and a cap early in the morning before work has been a perfect match for me. I now hate missing a swim and have so much more energy during my day. I'm much less stressed and I've even lost a few pounds. Exercising regularly has also motivated me to make better food choices. It all comes back to finding a form of exercise that worked for me.

Anything you do that elevates your heart rate, or uses more muscles more vigorously than you would during the rest of the day, is exercise — it's that simple! So whether you go to a gym, walk in the park or swim laps, you're doing exercise. And on days when you're feeling exhausted, a gentle exercise session of any type will probably make you feel better than either a hard workout or no exercise.

It's up to you whether you exercise in a gym, a local pool or simply walk or run in the park but always have a medical check-up before you start a vigorous exercise program. For example, suddenly taking up tennis if you're overweight and have a history of heart disease in your family could be more dangerous than healthy. It's also worth buying a heart rate monitor to check how intensely you're exercising.

Spontaneous exercise

Ten years ago, the average 30 to 40 year old did 5.5 miles more incidental or spontaneous exercise just

Your lifestyle	Suggested solution
High work stress affecting home life	Vigorous workout at the end of the day Duration: 20–30 minutes a day Intensity: heart rate above 140BPM but less than 200BPM minus your age
Limited time and excess weight	Exercise before breakfast Duration: 60–90 minutes a day Intensity: Low heart rate around 120–130BPM
Low serotonin levels	Exercise outside, especially in the sun Duration: 20 minutes a day Intensity: moderate — about 140BPM.
Trouble sleeping	Exercise outdoors in the middle of the day Duration: up to 90 minutes a day Intensity: moderate — about 140BPM
Unfocused with daily highs and lows of energy	Resistance training Duration: 20–45 minutes, three time a week Intensity: perform each exercise to fatigue

moving around in the course of daily life. As a society we are physically slowing down and mentally speeding up. So to stay naturally high with this increased mental pressure you need to stay physically active. Build movement into your everyday life — take the stairs, rather than the escalator; walk rather than drive and, if you do drive, park the car further away from your destination; get off the bus a few stops early and walk the rest of the way.

Vigorous walking for health

Frequent walking can make you very healthy and increase serotonin levels, but will not necessarily make you fit. Fitness requires that you increase your anaerobic threshold and the only way you can do this is to huff and puff a bit. Walking will lower blood pressure, decrease cholesterol and improve circulation but, unless you walk for longer than an hour each time, it doesn't move much body fat.

Rhythmic exercise to make you naturally high

When you rock a baby the rhythmic motion is very soothing, and gentle rhythmic exercise in children and adults has been shown to increase serotonin.

Swimming laps is an excellent rhythmic form of exercise that's been thought to increase serotonin. You can alternate between vigorous and gentler sessions, aiming to swim a total of about five times per week.

Exercise for deeper sleep

Exercise is an activity that produces more of your sleep chemical melatonin. This helps you achieve a deep sleep and gives your body a chance to make any required adaptations. So, if you're having trouble sleeping, you may find exercise helps you sleep deeply and wake up with a natural high.

Exercising puts a load or strain on the muscles — your neural pathways have to work in new ways and your ligaments and tendons are put under new stresses. Each time you exercise your body has to adapt to these added loads with most of this adaptation occurring as you sleep.

Exercise to raise your stress threshold

Your stress threshold is closely linked to how good you are at getting oxygen through the walls of your lungs and into your bloodstream. The anaerobic threshold is the point where the lungs can't extract more oxygen out of the air you breathe. Running, swimming or playing sports to the point where you're just out of breath will all improve your anaerobic threshold. As a result, everyday activities, which may have previously caused you to be out of breath, will become easy and fall under your threshold. You'll have more energy, be able to handle situations that demand high amounts of energy, recover more quickly from stress and strenuous activity, and generally feel more capable during the day. You can increase your threshold at any time in your life — in fact, the older you are the more you'll notice a change in how easy everyday activities become.

If you find the need to be naturally high on demand, two to four challenging workouts a week will pay off. A challenging workout stretches your comfort zone by pushing your oxygen system to work harder than it's used to. It's important to step up the pace progressively. If you walk a set route each day and it takes you 55 minutes, shave off a minute or two each week. On a stationary bike you may aim that by the end of the month you burn off another 50 calories in the same amount of time. It's the small changes over a week or so that cause your body to adapt and get stronger.

Finish vigorous workouts at the gym with five to ten minutes of gentler, winding down activities, for example walking on the treadmill at an easy pace with no incline, while breathing slowly and deeply. Follow this with a thorough, all over stretch program, and a shower before you go back to work or back home.

If you're suffering from stress you also need to address the environmental issues causing the stress, because if you don't address the cause of the stress, a day or so after the exercise your cortisol levels will creep back up and you'll need another fix of tough exercise. You could also become addicted to exercise and unable to feel good without it. While there are worse things to be addicted to, if you become addicted to exercise you'll be unable to feel good without it and you might go on exercising even when you need to stop. It's important not to exercise if you have the flu or a sore knee — when you're unwell you should rest for a day or so and give your body the time it needs to heal itself.

Resistance training to stabilize blood sugar

A regular resistance training program, for example body building, weight training or simple weight-bearing calisthenics (such as push-ups and bench dips), evens out blood sugar levels so you feel "up" more often during the day. Weight training is not just for men — women who weight train are also able to control body fat levels more easily, eat more of what they want and stay structurally strong. Whether you're a man or a woman, you probably don't want to become huge like Arnold Schwarzenegger. For the average person this isn't attainable without years of hard work and perhaps the help of drugs. But the unfounded fear of becoming huge and muscle bound may be preventing you from reaping the benefits of resistance training.

Through natural atrophy (wasting) everyone loses .5 pound of muscle every year after the age of 25. With resistance training you can halt and reverse this depreciation — you don't need to get big and muscle bound, you simply need to use your muscles. Resistance training also increases your metabolism by adding a little more muscle tissue. Muscle requires energy to stay alive — by adding 3 pounds of muscle tissue you'll increase your energy expenditure by 100 calories per day. Over one year this could add up to 36500 calories, which equates to about 11 pounds of fat.

One of the reasons you get tired and have days where energy levels go up and down is your inability to control the amount of insulin dumped by the pancreas from eating too much sugar. You body either dumps too much and you end up sleepy or it doesn't dump enough and you become hyperactive.

New findings have established that by increasing muscle mass people with diabetes have better control of their insulin and sugar responses. New research has shown that by increasing muscle mass by 2 to 4.5 pounds, type 2 diabetics were better able to manage sugar levels naturally.

In the early stages of resistance training the goal is simply to use your muscles more vigorously than they're used to. Once you get into it there are many variations depending on your goals. For example, in a gymnasium you could do a circuit of 10 to 20 exercise machines performing about 15 to 20 movements or repetitions and resting for around 30 seconds between each exercise. Or you may choose to do 30 to 45 minutes of weights two or three times a week, lifting heavier amounts and performing fewer repetitions (say 8 to 12). After a year of basic training you could then begin to focus on these specific training methods.

Exercise and your current chemical profile

It is always worth investing your time in exercise. You may like to choose a type of workout based on your current chemical profile.

Adrenaline

An adrenaline junkie will instinctively want to do fast, challenging exercise that may not be the best thing for their chemical balance. While any exercise is better than nothing, if you have a high adrenaline profile save your adrenaline for life's high pressure moments. Focus on continuous activity in preference to adrenaline-pumping high intensity. Rather than mountain biking, choose a steady ride away from traffic. Rather than boxing bouts, choose some bag and ball work. Again, aim for a steady level of intensity than the stop-start of a sparring session.

Serotonin

If you have a serotonin profile you may enjoy repetitive patterns and rhythmic movements. This includes swimming laps, walking a set route or working out on a rowing machine. You could even try kayaking early in the morning when it's calm and still and you can get a pattern going in your stroke. The key is to choose a mild intensity that you can maintain for at least 30 minutes. Don't start out hard only to run out of steam in 10 or 15 minutes. If you exercise first thing in the morning, you will help your body to switch off melatonin and switch on serotonin, securing a great start to the day.

Cortisol

Vigorous exercise that stretches you and pushes you to exhaustion is the key to managing cortisol. This is best used in a reactive fashion at the end of a tough day. Imagine you are burning off all the cortisol as you work out. A word of caution here: you need to have a certain level of fitness before you begin to use vigorous exercise as a stress management tool. You could try 100 yard sprints against a stopwatch. Sprint 100 yards, then walk back and repeat this pattern for 20 to 30 minutes. Map out a circuit in your local park or backyard and combine rhythmic sessions with calisthenics for 20 to 30 minutes.

Melatonin

Any physical exercise will help you sleep better. If you exercise in the middle of the day out in the sunshine, you get the double whammy of sunlight on the pineal gland and exercise elevating your melatonin levels. A walk in the park at lunchtime is ideal.

Insulin

Adding lean muscle tissue allows your body to control excess insulin. Weights, circuit training and calisthenics three times a week or every other day can help you achieve this. It's recommended to start weight training with some supervision, so employ a trainer for one or two sessions or join a gym with a free introductory program as part of the membership. You need to be pretty familiar with weight training movements before you set up a home gym.

getting the most out of exercise

Eating before exercise

If you exercise on an empty stomach you'll use more fat than you would normally — because your blood sugar is low your body can't easily get its energy from sugar. Overnight your metabolism slows down to its lowest ebb for the 24-hour period. During this 8 to 10 hour period you don't eat any more food — when you wake from this fasting your blood sugar is low. So going for a brisk walk before you "break your fast" means you'll use more fat as a fuel than you would exercising after eating.

But if you struggle to have the energy to exercise at the best of times, eat something before you start. The extra amount of fat burned by not having anything to eat may be offset by a lackluster effort due to hunger and fatigue. If you can stomach it, eat and then work a little harder. For example, eating a banana will get some quickly digested sugar into your bloodstream, giving your body an easy energy source for the exercise.

Minimizing tiredness

You may find you need to go to bed earlier on the days you exercise. Your body uses the sleep to repair damage to muscle tissues and strengthen them for the next time you exercise. So you may be tired because you need more sleep.

Food timing may also been causing the tiredness. If you eat within 30 minutes of finishing exercise, and eat the medium to high glycemic index foods, you'll be able to increase your body's energy supplies.

Do quality exercise before quantity

When exercising, always do quality before quantity. For most people, a little cardiovascular work, such as riding a bike, walking on a treadmill or participating in an aerobics class, will act as a warm-up for resistance training. But depending on your exercise goals, you may want to switch the order.

If you're seriously getting into resistance training to sculpt your body, improve strength or for injury-rehabilitation, you need to work when you're fresh. The idea is to put quality before quantity and do your weights before your cardio. Start with a short 10 minute warm-up to get the blood pumping and then do your weight program. Be sure to do a few light warm-up sets before each exercise. Afterward you can do a cardiovascular session, if you feel like it.

Research has shown that doing weights, particularly for the lower body, depletes your muscle sugars and, like the pre-breakfast workout, gives you a chance to burn more fat later when you jump on the stairclimber or walk that killer hill three times.

Churchill's urge

Exercise is a wonderful body-balancing tool. Easy exercise elevates serotonin levels and vigorous or tough exercise breaks down cortisol. Regular exercise increases your ability to handle pressure and changes your mood. Exercising for an hour every day is an investment that reaps returns in your other 23 hours. You'll sleep better, digest food more easily, relax more quickly and have an increased focus at work.

1 Regular exercise lays a foundation for peak performance, giving you more energy, improving stress thresholds and burning up stress chemicals.

2 Vigorous or tough workouts are most effective for improving fitness and energy levels, as well as temporarily lowering adrenaline levels.

3 Gentle rhythmic workouts raise serotonin levels, as well as burn fat and lower cholesterol levels.

4 Regular exercise allows you to elevate your stress threshold so you can manage greater crises without losing your equilibrium.

lights

5 Resistance training to build lean muscle tissue helps moderate insulin responses and manage high sugar hits.

If I look confused it's

because I'm thinking.

SAMUEL GOLDWYN

9

mind over matter

thinking differently

I guess I was stuck in a rut — the safety of a salary meant I didn't have to bet on myself. I've always wanted to run my own business but lacked the confidence. "What if I fail?" "How will I feed my family?" As a single mom my sense of responsibility was huge. I would get into a spiral of doubt often searching my daily life for evidence that I couldn't make it. Of course I found heaps of evidence for why going it alone can cost you everything — you really do find what you seek! I would read bankruptcy case studies and talk to anyone who had a story of small business failure! The more I indulged in this negative thinking and problem finding, the more depressed I got. So it came as no surprise that my work performance began to decrease — everything seemed to be unraveling. When the layoffs came I was more or less forced to take a severance and make it work. Necessity is a great motivator and now that I'm running my own show I'm working harder than I ever did for an employer. I have gradually built the business over the last three years and, while there are anxious moments, I take faith in my success so far and give myself a good talking to. I'm much more confident now about my own ability and realize that most of my fears were manufactured in my own head. What a waste of time! I don't think I would let myself spiral into such a negative thought pattern again. It didn't help — all I did was lose sleep, hurt friends and live in a self-made psychological hell.

Feeling high is as much psychological as it is chemical: your thoughts and chemistry are inextricably linked. When you balance your thoughts you balance your chemistry. Although changing how you think is less tangible than changing your diet, exercise and sleeping patterns, it's equally important.

SNAPSHOT

Adrenaline plays a large part in your behavior if you find others are too slow for you and you are quite decisive.

Serotonin plays a large part in your behavior if you pause before acting.

Cortisol makes you anxious and uptight and is probably the fuel for most negative thought habits.

Lack of sleep means you'll play out your worst behaviors or the stress version of your personality. Melatonin is the key to deep sleep.

With either too much or too little sugar it's hard to think straight. Insulin regulates this delicate balance.

success momentum

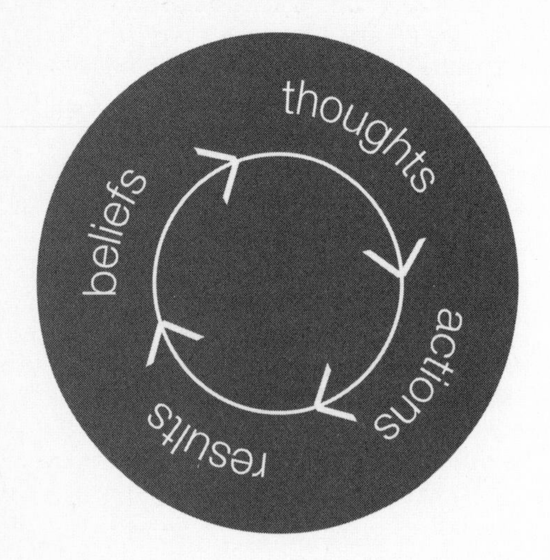

Control your thoughts and your chemistry will follow — an empowering concept. Choose clarity over chaos and your adrenal system will be there when an important challenge arises. Choose happiness over depression, or optimism over helplessness, and your serotonin system will back you up. Choose calm over anxiety and you'll prevent your cortisol system from taking over. Choose when and what to eat and insulin will become an ally, increasing your mental focus rather than making you slow, sluggish or sleepy. Developing patterns and habits around when you sleep and what you think about before you go to bed all help you balance melatonin and sleep more effectively.

To change your thought processes, or unlearn old ways of thinking, you need two things — responsibility and optimism. You must avoid personal blame yet take responsibility for your part in the problem. And you must hold on to a certain hope that things will get better — these are the principles of cognitive psychotherapy.

Feeling naturally high means taking responsibility for changing what you can about your life that's making you unhappy. At the same time you need to be optimistic that every day, through a constant focus on improvement, you can make things better. By doing this over time, you build success momentum — you have a thought and take action, which provides a result that then reinforces a belief, which in turn affects future thoughts.

changing habits

If you can learn a habit, like picking up a bowl, you can learn or even unlearn other thought habits. You can also choose to think differently. The process is the same; first you need to become conscious of a certain thought pattern and then you have to take steps to do things differently. After a while this becomes habit and your chemistry will follow suit.

When you lift your arm a miracle occurs. At four to six months old you began to notice this thing called a hand, which often waved in and out of your vision. One day after eating some banana you realized that quite by accident you could knock things over with your hand. For a while you observed in amazement

The power of the mind

Frequent double blind studies using real medications and placebos (a sugar pill containing no medication) have shown that a percentage of those taking the placebo had effective results. In a study of the anti nausea drug ondansetron hydrochloride, 96% of those who took the real drug said it was effective — 10% of those on the placebo also reported effectiveness. Those taking the sugar pills believed they must be taking the real medication and so it worked for them — the power of the mind over the body.

that as you looked at the bowl of banana the hand moved toward it. A realization of self had begun. Through repetition and a process of discovery you connected that the hand was a part of you and that you could influence where it went and what it did. Each time you moved the hand and connected with the bowl you were reinforcing the thought and motor skill of banging. Over time a clumsy knock of the bowl evolved into a layer of complex skills like sticking your hand in the banana, wiping the banana on your father's new dress shirt and so on.

four stages of learning

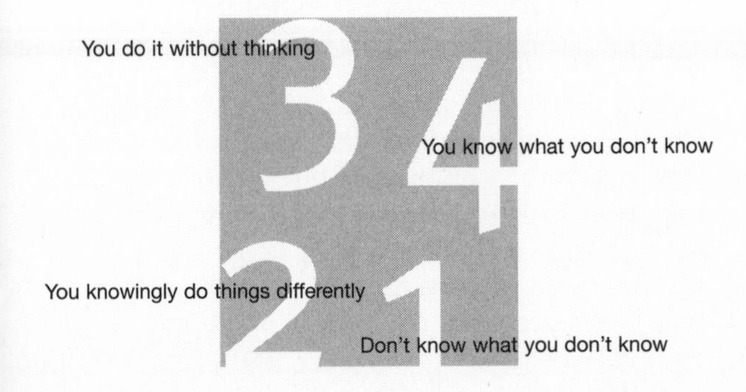

Neural pathways are activated at these early stages of growth and through constant use and mental reinforcement a habit begins. This phenomenon continues through the rest of your life — you learn something quite consciously and then it eventually becomes habit.

the chemistry of thought

Thoughts can affect your chemical balance profile in profound ways. For example, when you're asleep you may have a nightmare which causes obvious physical changes — you sweat and your body pumps adrenaline and cortisol. And when you lose a loved one you go through a grieving process that causes low serotonin and leads to depression.

Author of *Learned Optimism* and a leading researcher into cognitive therapy, Martin Selegman, believes it's possible to think yourself happy. It's true that thoughts are affected by your chemistry but it's equally possible you can think unhappy thoughts as a result of too few "feel good" chemicals in your system.

As you read this there's an internal dialogue going on between your ears. If you're thinking "No there isn't," you've just proved my point. This chatter becomes so customary it's easily forgotten. The language of your inner voice is the key to understanding your thoughts — your internal dialogue and the words you speak out loud reflect what state your mind is in and in turn this reflects your chemical balance profile.

obstacles to getting what you want

If you haven't been able to get what you want in life, it could be because:

1 you don't know what you want
2 you don't know how to get what you want
3 someone or something is in the way.

Goal setting and dreaming is the key to overcoming the first. There are many courses and books on setting goals. Reading self-help books or attending seminars is also how you deal with the second. Read a book on the five steps to weight loss and you get a strategy of sorts, you now have an idea of how to get what you want. It's the third obstacle that many people get stuck on.

Often the someone who's in the way is you! Whether you're a born negative thinker or have become so because of your environment is the nature versus nurture discussion. But whether nature or nurture is responsible isn't relevant — you are what you are right now and simply need to do the best you can with what you have. You can change your circumstances — you have to want to and you must believe you can make a difference. But you can do it.

adrenaline junkies — clear your mind

If you're an adrenaline junkie, you're a decisive quick thinker, able to focus on more than one thing at a time. You're highly self-motivated, passionate and confident.

But you can come across as uncaring and ungrateful. You demand so much of yourself that you often forget to thank others for their contributions and in your haste you disconnect from people and lose your sense of priority.

Have you ever had a thought just as you begin to fall asleep? A nagging reminder of what you forgot to do and need to finish the next day. That's how I used to be all the time — my head always full of things I needed to do. I had never been taught how to organize my thoughts. Looking back I don't know how I didn't self-destruct. I had left school early and got straight into work — if it had been around at the time I think I might have been diagnosed with hyperactive attention deficit disorder when I was a kid. I'm proud of all that I've accomplished in my life but realize now I've moved ahead in life by throwing more energy at it than others are willing to — my energy is still legendary at work and I pride myself on working as hard, if not harder, than any of my staff. The fashion industry is all about passion so it helps to have plenty.

But I found that a few simple organizational skills have freed me up to balance work and life, while still achieving great things at work. I now write lists, plan my projects in advance and use a diary — I'd be lost without my Daytimer! I also carry a creative ideas journal with me — so now rather than loose bits of paper and loose thoughts I have a log book of ideas, sketches of new designs and a shorthand of what was agreed to in nearly every meeting I attend.

An adrenaline junkie who's organized is a force to be reckoned with! Known for your prodigious energy, you can go so fast your head simply overloads as you fuel your need for speed by handling more and more tasks. Although having a lot going on is exciting, clearing your mind and developing organizational tools gives direction to your energy. You still go fast but now at least you're facing in the right direction.

Slow down your thoughts

It's sometimes easier to go fast through life so you don't have to stop and think too much about what's really important.

Under stress most people go faster — for an adrenaline junkie speed is the preferred response to most things. You say, "There are never enough hours in the day to do all I want." To say you want too much is limiting because of course you want it all, or at least a good go at getting it.

But you do need to question your belief that speed is right and instead aim for more haste and less speed.

The current trend in society of instant gratification has led to a speed addiction, but this worship of fast sometimes diminishes the quality of life and relationships.

So slow down your thoughts from time to time and have deep and long thoughts rather than quick and shallow ones.

Do less to have more

The thoughts you fill your head with don't always help you get more of what you want in life. So get all your thoughts working toward what's important and dump the rest. Don't look for more to satisfy you. Less could be what you're looking for, in fact.

Systemize the mundane

In an attempt to be busy and stay on adrenaline you may be using up unnecessary headspace on mundane activities that could be managed automatically and effectively through systems.

A story goes that a visiting professor at an academic function asks Einstein for his telephone number so he can call to discuss further his theory of relativity. Einstein off-handedly replies that he doesn't know his own number. In jest the professor scoffs at him at first and then asks incredulously, "How could one of the world's greatest intelligences not know his own number?," to which Einstein replies, "When would I need to ever call myself? And if for some reason I did have the need, I know I could look up my number in the telephone directory. So I choose not to fill my head with information I could find elsewhere."

Edward de Bono, the man who coined the term "lateral thinking," saves head space by going through the same procedure each time he leaves a hotel room. He still checks every drawer (even though he knows he didn't unpack his bag) then goes through the bathroom tossing all the towels into the bathtub to make sure nothing of his has become caught up in them. By following this procedure every time he is able to think about other things on the way to the airport, confident he left nothing personal behind.

Think about how you're wasting head space and develop systems and habits to avoid wasting thoughts or time on the mundane.

Avoid speed talking and speed thinking
When you say you're flat out busy and don't have enough time to get everything done, you reaffirm a lack. Using and thinking words and phrases like "urgent" or "as soon as possible" will hurry everything up. Not everything needs to be quick.

Constant speed talking and speed thinking will eventually cause adrenal fatigue. So watch your thought processes and what you say — check whether you're affirming a lack of time just to feel busy and keep "on" adrenaline.

Adjust your thought time lines
When running on adrenaline you risk becoming a time line thinker. When feeling negative you dwell on the past and when feeling positive you're future focused — thoughts of what's coming up tomorrow, chasing a vision, goal or objective. Becoming present in the now is a Zen concept and totally appropriate for adrenaline junkies.

Connect to what's happening right now around you. Take a moment to hear the noises and observe the colors and textures of what's within reach. Be here now.

serotonin seekers — think good thoughts

If you're a serotonin seeker you're highly attuned to the needs of others — you're caring and focused on comfort. Sensitive to your environment, you're capable of feeling deeply and are usually creative.

But you can be oversensitive, magnifying problems out of proportion, which may stop you getting what you want in life. If you're not a good communicator, anger or anxiety may be the result.

I don't know what got hold of me last week. It was as if my thoughts weren't my own. I had missed a few nights' sleep and it had been raining for days — being stuck indoors always gives me cabin fever. Anyway, I became paranoid and started manufacturing problems that, thinking back, had no foundation in reality. I took every comment personally and almost lost my sense of humor. That changed almost overnight. There's a comedy club near my home and a friend somehow convinced me to go there one night. I'm so glad I did! Initially I wasn't looking forward to it because I find most live comedians use too much swearing in their humor. This night they had all accepted the challenge to tell clean jokes — I had a ball. It was such a tonic for me and I walked out having laughed for 3 hours straight. It gave me a new perspective on everything.

Because I had begun to lose my sense of humor everything took on a greater meaning. I was suffering from stinking thinking — my thoughts certainly needed a good wash!

Your mission as a serotonin seeker is to think good thoughts about yourself and to defend against irrational thoughts, which sabotage your calm. You need to ask yourself: "How does this make me feel? Is that a rational thought? Is that just a feeling, or is it a fact? What can I do to change this situation?"

Defending your self-esteem is critical. With high self-esteem you can make the lifestyle choices that nourish you and balance your chemistry. Good self-esteem comes from a positive self-image (your personal belief about what you deserve to get in life), good self-worth (how much you value yourself) and healthy self-confidence (how comfortable you feel putting yourself and opinions up for evaluation and feedback).

Your self image is largely formed from the beliefs others had for you — if you had an upbringing that encouraged you to believe you could be everything you wanted to be you're likely to have fewer limiting beliefs about your potential. What you think you have to offer others is a good measure of your self worth. For example, people with a high self-worth will see themselves in meetings as having something to contribute. If your ideas are listened to and valued your self-worth increases. But if every time you pipe up you aren't taken seriously, feelings of low self-worth develop. If you lack self-confidence you'll tend to sit quietly in groups or meetings, feeling that although you might have faith in your opinions you don't want to risk being judged. This is a fear that eventually steals your self-worth and alters your self-image.

Maintain a sense of humor

When you're feeling down and dealing with serious life issues, maintaining a sense of humor can be difficult.

If you think a joke is an attempt to criticize you or devalue you in the eyes of others, you'll take the joke to heart. But by taking the light humor to heart you allow the joker to steal a small piece of your self-worth. You can't change people or their comments, you can only change your response to them. If your self-esteem is high you'll take a chance comment from someone else in good humor.

Develop thoughts of your own about your worthiness — the favor of others then becomes less important.

Educate yourself

Learning broadens your thinking and helps you develop behavioral flexibility.

One of the best ways to educate yourself, and therefore build self-esteem, is to ask questions and become well read. They say that if you were to build a pile of what humankind knows today, within three years the pile will have doubled. All you need to do to keep up and have an opinion is to read. Don't worry if you feel sometimes you're overloading your brain and not retaining what you read, hear and see — assimilation is a process of saturation.

You can also listen to audio tapes in the car or at the gym, attend seminars, or attend a night-time course. Consider going back to college and begin educating yourself in your areas of weakness.

Build others up

The more you do to build others up, the more your own self-image skyrockets. It also helps your chemical balance profile. Self-centered thinking, on the other hand, encourages you to dwell on problems and blow things out of proportion.

You can specifically build someone else up by avoiding criticism and being a good listener, giving them your full attention. When you praise someone, be specific. Focusing your thoughts on others helps you avoid the self-indulgent thinking of an out-of-balance adrenaline junkie or serotonin seeker.

Spend time with a variety of people

If you always hang around the same type of people you risk rigid thinking.

Think differently by mixing with different types of people. Strive to avoid the cliques and groups that form out of people's need to be with others like them; instead get involved in your community and volunteer for committees. Begin to think about diversity and you'll be less likely to abuse one chemical over another.

stinking thinking

Rigid thinking, selective thinking and blowing out are poor thinking habits that can sabotage your chance of success and are common problems for both adrenaline junkies and serotonin seekers.

Rigid thinking

Rigid, all-or-nothing thinking is what leads to racism, intolerance and pigheadedness. This kind of thinking allows for only one way and leads to a chemical imbalance.

Words like "never" and "always" abound when you fall into rigid thinking. You judge yourself harshly, have unrealistic expectations and set yourself up for failure by "musts" and "shoulds," shouldn'ts" and "oughts" — it's as if you need to be whipped and punished before you could be expected to do anything. The emotional consequence is guilt and when you direct these statements toward others you feel anger, resentment or frustration.

Soften the judgments on yourself and others, and make room for greater flexibility.

Selective thinking

When you think selectively you put on a mental filter that picks out a single negative detail and dwells on it exclusively, regardless of tangible positive signs to the contrary. You arbitrarily conclude that someone is reacting negatively to you, and don't bother to check this out. Anticipating that things will turn out badly, you feel convinced that your prediction is an already established fact. By converting every positive experience into a negative one you often become cynical.

Like the drop of ink that discolors a beaker of water, your vision of all reality becomes darkened. For example, if your performance falls short of perfect, you see yourself as a total failure. And you'll also see other people as either fabulous or failures. You may even see yourself as the cause of some negative external event which you were not primarily responsible for.

Focusing on the negative also means you reject positive experiences by insisting that they "don't count" for some reason or other — in this way you can maintain a belief that's contradicted by your everyday experiences. You assume that your negative emotions necessarily reflect the way things are: "I feel it, therefore it must be true." If you make a mistake, you attach a negative label to yourself, such as "I'm a loser," and when someone else's behavior rubs you the wrong way, you attach a negative label to him or her such as "He's a goddamn louse" — this is mislabeling an event by describing it in highly colored and emotionally loaded language.

In its extreme, selective thinking creates a gulf between you and others. You can feel resentment toward the great things others have in their life and begin to see yourself as unlucky or jinxed.

Break this thought habit by developing an attitude of gratitude. Start listing what's good in your life and acknowledging praise genuinely. It also helps to develop a complimentary style in your interaction with others, but be careful to avoid comparative compliments such as "You're so good at sports, I've never been able to play team sports." If you have trouble praising others because it feels insincere, develop the practice of specific praise. Focus exactly on what you admire in their behavior.

Blowing out

Blowing out is catastrophic thinking where you exaggerate the importance of things, or inappropriately shrink them until they appear tiny (also called the binocular trick).

It's easy to take a negative situation and make it worse by exaggerating it in your mind, particularly if you see a single negative event as a never ending pattern of defeat. If you're realistic you know that not everything in life is going to be rosy all the time. Continual positive thinking in the face of obvious negatives is just another form of unrealistic thinking, but when you blow out a problem and make it bigger than it really is, your thinking has become distorted. For example, you might generalize everything ("This always happens to me"), or exaggerate the problem into a catastrophe ("What if the train is derailed?"). You may even personalize every situation ("She gave me a strange look, I must look weird").

Thinking investment portfolio

1. Plan more often and react less
2. Eat more often and crave less
3. Drink more water and thirst less
4. Pause more often and spin out less
5. Workout more and be worn out less
6. Communicate more often and guess less

Break the thought habit of blowing out by putting things in perspective, keeping a sense of humor and gathering facts before jumping to conclusions. Adjust language such as "always," "never" and "catastrophic" to soften the suggestion that there's no way out of a situation. Ask yourself, "Will this really matter when I'm 80 years old?" to bring things into perspective.

It's also important to stay open — sometimes you can blow out with others by never giving them a second chance ("She disagreed with me in that meeting so I'm never going to support her").

mind over matter

Your thoughts and current chemical balance profile work hand in hand. If you think negative distorted thoughts, your body will support that process and lower your serotonin. If you're always speed thinking, your body will dump more adrenaline. Choosing how you think balances your chemistry and is a powerful contributor to a naturally high life.

highlights

1 Feeling high is as much psychological as it is chemical. Understanding how you think will help you choose a higher life.

2 Thought habits teach your chemistry how to behave. You can learn new habits and unlearn those that don't help balance your body chemistry.

3 By looking within and determining what thoughts are not helpful, you become conscious of what you want to change and can then find out how to make those changes. Over time these new ways of thinking become habitual.

4 Adrenaline junkies need to clear thought clutter and serotonin seekers need to eliminate bad thoughts.

5 The three common stinking thinking habits of rigid thinking, selective thinking and blowing out can develop regardless of your current chemical balance profile.

10

high stress

> Future shock is the shattering stress and disorientation that we induce in individuals by subjecting them to too much change in too short a time.
>
> ALVIN TOFFLER

good and bad stress

Working for a computer software company by day and doing consulting at night means time is at a premium. My two eldest boys from my previous marriage are now in college — I'm proud of all my children and wanted to help them financially as much as I could but I started stressing about money. Josh, my third boy, needed some major dental work, which made a big hole in my bank account. On top of that, tension was building with my ex-wife as my job meant I was frequently away, often on weekends, which resulted in having to change visitation weekends at short notice.

My wife and I recently found out our five-year-old daughter has autism. I knew my wife really needed me, but with the travel and working two jobs I was smothered. I find it hard to say "no" to people and I knew we needed extra money to pay for therapists for Nicole — I wanted to give her the best opportunities. Of course I ended up overcommitting myself and spread myself so thin I didn't feel I was giving any part of my life my best. Diet and exercise didn't even get a moment's notice.

Then I got a scare when I discovered my cholesterol was through the roof. I did a stress test that week and the doctors found unusual heart rhythms. This was the wake-up call. I started saying "no" to non-essential tasks and negotiated more work from home with less travel. I also made sure I had at least three healthy meals a day. I have more energy now, my performance has improved significantly and of course my families are also benefiting.

Stress is the damage caused by an unbalanced use of your body chemistry. Although the causes vary between individuals, the results are the same. Switching on adrenaline to cope with crisis or to perform well is great. Leaving it switched on is stress. A natural high needs the calm relaxed state of serotonin as well as adrenaline — when you're stressed you can end up stuck on adrenaline.

But stress is not all bad. A little stress helps you stretch, grow and expand your comfort zones — it can provide the stimulus of challenge for optimum functioning.

The up side of stress

Mental alertness is increased
Social obligations are met
Physical strength for emergencies is summoned
Love and affection is won
Growth is nurtured
Creativity is stimulated

The down side of stress

Stomach problems
Chronic skin troubles
Heart disease
Tension headaches
Obesity
Mental breakdowns
Kidney problems
High blood pressure
Colitis

SNAPSHOT

Adrenaline is released when you're challenged in any way.

High serotonin increases the ability to handle change and pressure.

Constant stress increases cortisol levels, resulting in greater anxiety, irritability and a loss of calm.

Negatively influencing melatonin levels, constant stress hinders sleep.

Cravings for sugar increase under stress, causing excessive insulin release and resulting in drowsiness and poor focus.

It's constant stress, or stress that's too great, that creates a natural low. High stress can also cause serious physical and psychological harm. World-renowned stress expert Dr. Hans Selye refers to good stress as "eustress" as opposed to health destroying "distress." Eustress and distress are not in fact different things — they are the same physical response, and can be caused by the same life events. What determines whether it's stimulation or strain is simply whether the stress is too intense, or goes on for too long, for your body to handle. Stress is inevitable; burning out is not — distinguishing between the two is how you determine whether you're stressed or simply busy. The point at which eustress becomes distress is different for each individual.

high breaking points

With three children, a busy private practice and an elderly mother suffering from Alzheimer's it hasn't been easy. My eldest daughter is doing her SAT this year and my sister and I have also had some tense moments and disagreements over Mom's care. It's very painful watching my mother's health deteriorate when she used to be such an alert and energetic woman, but I've managed not to fall apart. I think what has helped is acknowledging that this is stressful and allowing time to myself. I do regular deep relaxation and yoga in the evenings with my children and exercise during my lunch break. I also make sure I have some fun time with the children — not just chores and homework and getting them to school on time.

Everyone experiences stress at some stage, from moving or getting married, to professional landmarks and career challenges. Some of these events are welcome, and some not — all are challenging and demand time and energy. Over time, you may be affected by a number of stressful events, some long-term and some short-lived. And at different times, you may find your stress level being pushed over your threshold.

You've probably noticed that some people seem to sail through these events, while others fall apart at the first signs of difficulty. This is because everyone has a different stress threshold, or how much stress you can handle before it begins to affect your health or performance. Stressful events can add up.

For example, if two people, Jill and Sally, both face a series of three challenges in their life, each one of greater impact than the last, they will hit their stress thresholds at different times.

Both Sally and Jill will cope with Event A with no problem. Similarly, Event C will overwhelm them both

stress threshold

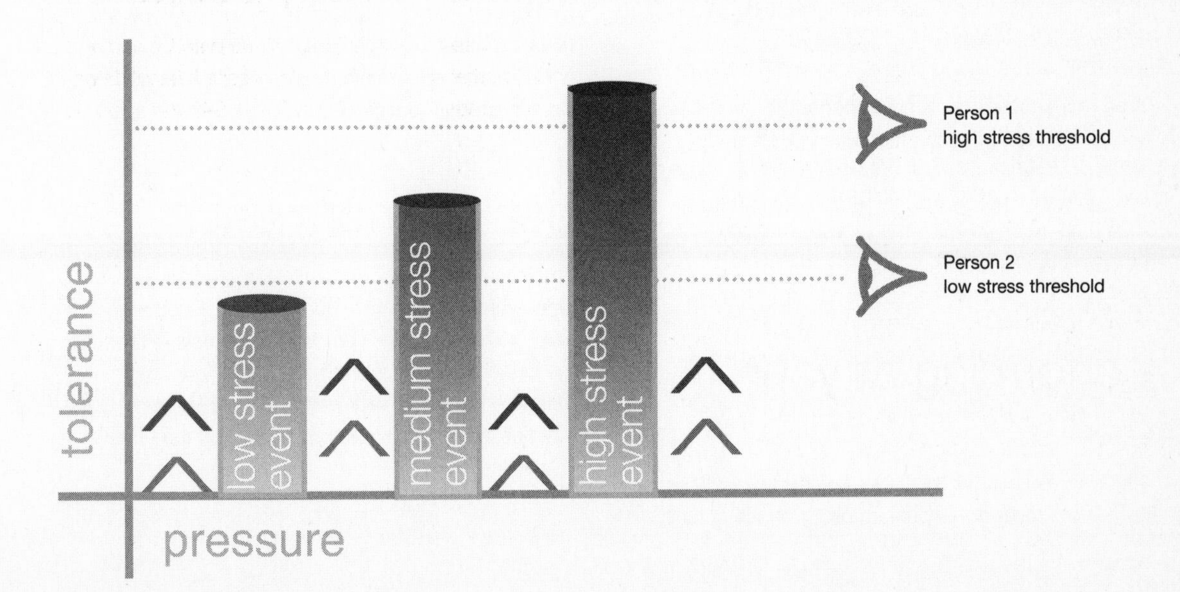

if they don't get help. The difference between Sally and Jill will be obvious only in Event B — the one with which Jill will cope and which Sally will find highly stressful.

There are only two moments where the stress threshold is exceeded — Event C. Sally and Jill both deal with the greatest single stress, right at the end of the diagram, because it's isolated. The earlier events wouldn't have been a problem except for the long-term, low-level stress which added to them.

Melting point

Regardless of how high your stress threshold is, you can still suffer from burnout. You have the capacity to take on more and more pressure until one day it hits you — the pressure comes in so many forms that it's often hard to identify the particular activities creating the stress. It's tempting to blame the event that pushed you over the edge when actually it's an accumulation of events over several days.

Time management skills are important to avoid piling stresses on top of each other. Eating well, getting regular moderate exercise, thinking positively, getting enough sleep, taking downtime and doing regular relaxation practice all raise your stress threshold as well as increase energy levels.

performing at your peak

Although you might think there are only two options — flat out or stopped — optimum performance actually comes about not from being relaxed, or from being highly aroused, but somewhere in between. Arousal refers to the state of brain and body activity — ranging from totally relaxed to totally aroused. Matching arousal to the task and matching the task to the level of skill appear to be the keys to entering the mental state of peak performance, known in sports as the flow state or "the zone."

If the task is too easy or too hard, the athlete will generally not experience the zone and performance won't flow. If the task is within the athlete's level of skill, but still hard enough to make them stretch themself, they may experience the zone. This is not only effective, but also pleasurable, a natural high. Athletes describe this state with phrases such as "the performance just seemed to happen."

One of the major focuses of sports psychology is teaching athletes to manage their level of arousal to achieve peak performance, sometimes referred to as the "inverted U" principle.

peak performance

Arousal increases your speed, strength and reaction time, while it decreases your precision, control and ability to reason. The more familiar you are with a task, the higher the level of arousal you can use, and therefore the better your performance. The more you practice, the more familiar you'll be with the task.

optimal arousal

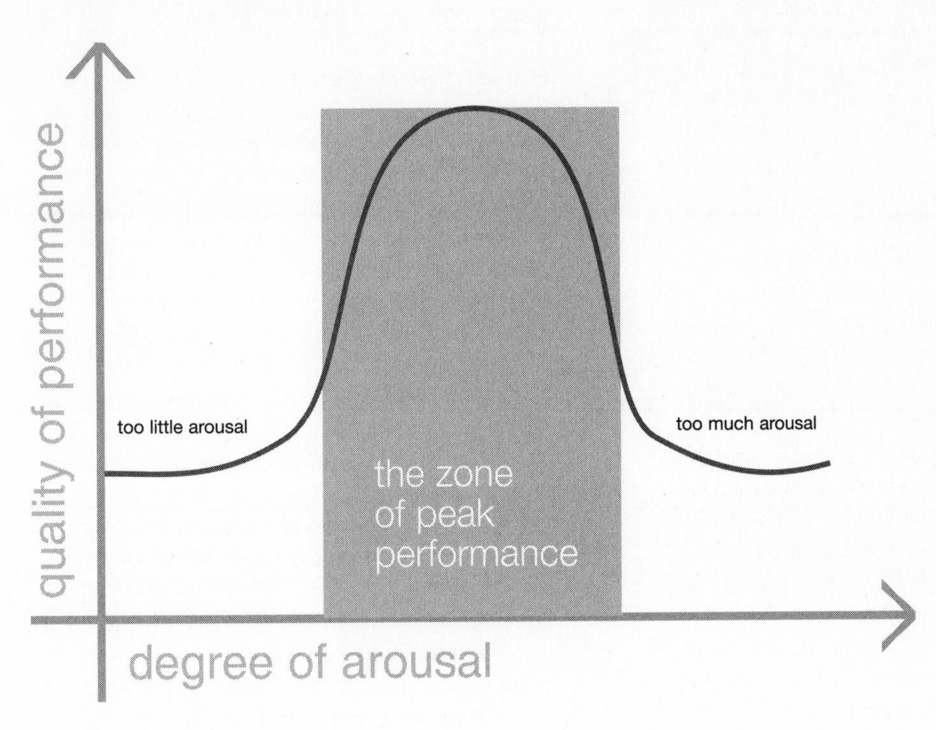

For peak performance, higher levels of arousal are needed for tasks that are:

- more physical
- familiar to you
- relatively simple
- less precise
- of shorter duration

For peak performance, lower levels of arousal are needed for tasks that are:

- more cognitive
- less familiar to you
- complex
- require precision
- longer in duration

Stressed or simply busy?

1. Would you describe yourself as energetic?
2. Are you clear on what to do when your working day comes to an end?
3. Do you have a lot to say to people?
4. Are you taking vacations to discover new things (as opposed to vacations to recover)?
5. Can you find joy in the smallest thing?
6. Are you patient with those closest to you?
7. Are you seeing your family and friends as much as you would like?
8. Are you into sex at the moment (or is it more trouble than it's worth)?
9. Are you getting more and more done (or is your productivity dropping off?)
10. Do you regularly laugh at yourself?

If you answered "no" to 4 or more answers you're on the way to burnout.

Peaking early

I used to get so worked up before doing anything important — I wouldn't call it nerves so much as just excited. The problem was I peaked early. I would get into, say, the dinner party only to be exhausted half way through. I think that by spending the whole day looking forward to the night and thinking of all the things I wanted to talk about I simply ran out of energy. I've also noticed this at work. I try now to stay cool before I get into a long meeting or complex conversation. In the past I would plan the meeting in my head 10 times before I got there. Talk about overkill — I must have so much more head space now!

In anything you do, there is an optimal level of arousal. When peak performance is required, you need to use your high-performance, adrenaline-based system — and manage the rush (Adrenaline Priority Event). For example, professional speakers, athletes and entertainers need a degree of tension or arousal for a good performance. Such people sometimes report that learning relaxation techniques makes their performance worse. This is because of inappropriate use of relaxation.

Generally, if you're taking a test, the more relaxed you are the better. If you know the material thoroughly, a little more arousal may speed you up. But if you're uncertain, you need to relax and take your time, even though the less certain you are the more uptight you're likely to be.

Symptoms of over-arousal include verbal and physical clumsiness, a sense of disconnection from what's going on, inaccuracy and a sense of urgency or panic. You're under aroused if your performance is below its usual standards. You feel flat, uninspired or slow, you're not firing and perhaps don't really care. An adrenaline trigger may be what you need to raise your arousal, or perhaps you simply need rest because you're exhausted or burned out.

Slowing down the pace

1 Minimize the roller-coaster effect of rush and crash. When you find fear driving your life, or see yourself getting wound up, ask yourself "Do I need to be in a state of arousal or emergency for this?" Is this an Adrenaline Priority Event? Often the answer is "no."

2 Do mild exercise to burn off the adrenaline and cortisol. If you find you can't come down after a rush of adrenaline, exercise will also help.

3 Stop taking yourself and events around you so seriously. A sense of humor is one of the most effective ways to decrease your body's stress chemicals.

4 Force yourself to slow down. Place your hands on the table, take a deep breath and slow down the pace.

5 Get away from the stresses. Avoid eating lunch at your desk surrounded by the tools for productivity and piles of papers that remind you of what remains undone.

6 Connect to your environment. It's hard to maintain an adrenaline edge when you connect to the color of flowers, the smell of roasting coffee or the effect of wind on water. People's faces also allow you to focus on something outside your stimulators and get off the "merry-go-round."

7 Get away. Long weekends away from the hustle and bustle are ideal serotonin breaks. The vacation prescription may help you justify time off.

Vacation prescription:
6 long weekends every year
2 two-week vacations a year
and every 18 months to 3 years a 4–8 week break

the importance of downtime

To ensure a long, healthy and successful life you need to take downtime. When you deliberately relax, a series of chemical (brain and body) changes occur, which wind the body down (bringing it out of crisis preparation). This slows down many of the high-performance functions, and readies it for more mundane tasks such as digesting food, repairing tissue damage and fighting off illness. Your body is then able to replenish energy stores, increase serotonin and restore adrenaline.

This is the flow of nature — you're meant to have "highs" and "lows." In winter, bears slow down or hibernate — human physiology also has a winter slowdown when you sleep and eat more, and store more fat. You also have two low points during a 24 hour day, one between 3:00 and 4:00 a.m. and another between 3:00 and 4:00 p.m. The challenge is, modern society doesn't always allow for this slowdown — the shareholders' desire for profit doesn't take a couple of months off in winter.

Uptime means using the high arousal, adrenaline state to do what it does best — being alert and focused on the external world. It is interacting with others, focusing on your goal and performing at your best. Uptime is when you make things happen and is associated with the "rush." Provided you haven't burned yourself out through overuse of the adrenaline system, you don't generally need to do anything specific to switch into uptime mode.

Downtime is when you rebalance, enjoy time for yourself and allow serotonin levels to be restored. Your focus turns inward, and your attention is given to your own needs. If you're trying to be a peak performer you're probably under-using this system. While you try to stay in uptime, your body is craving downtime. Fighting this need is a losing battle — the secret of being "on" 80% of the time is being "off" 20% of the time.

If you're not used to doing this at all, it will take some practice to develop the skill to take downtime and relax. Regular deep relaxation practice will help you relax at will. And once your body relearns the relaxation response, you'll find you can trigger it easily with the following "circuit breaker" activities. Even if you don't do deep relaxation, the circuit breakers help you step away from over arousal. These can be done without anyone around you being aware you're doing them.

Take a brief pause

Turn your attention to your breath for a few minutes at a suitable pause in your activities. If you've been using the relaxation techniques regularly, you'll find your breath becomes a relaxation trigger. You can leave your eyes open while you do this, and remain aware of people around you. It's simply a "pulling back" for a time and allows the sense of urgency to depart. Also notice the physical tension you've been building up, and take a moment to drop your shoulders back where they should be. Then come back to alertness, switch back on and get on with the job. You'll find you last much longer by taking the occasional pause.

Enjoy meal times

Instead of working over a sandwich, take the time to notice what you're eating. Tune in to the aspects of your environment that you normally tune out while you're focused and working. Serotonin is not only associated with calmness, it's also connected to sensory awareness.

Indulge in non stressful activities

Make sure you occasionally indulge in activities that are not stressful, not career oriented, and that require you to have your awareness only in the present. This can include sports, chess or computer games. Reading a novel, or even taking a bath, are also options. Some people criticize these approaches as being ways of "escaping from reality." There's nothing wrong with an occasional escape, providing you're not using these methods to avoid doing what needs to be done.

the art of deep relaxation

Practicing deep relaxation will make your circuit breakers more effective. I recommend one or two sessions of deep relaxation, of 10 to 20 minutes duration daily. Ideally, schedule these sessions for the same time every day. For those who have 9 to 5 style careers, a midmorning and an after work session works well. In an open plan office a 10-minute meditation can be construed as thinking and in a way it is. The after work session (done as soon as you get home) can also help you separate work and home life. Even parking the car before you walk in, or sitting at the train station for a minute before you meet the kids, this time will make you more effective when you need to swing into child care.

Deep relaxation works best after exercise rather than before, when the body is winding down anyway. Avoid deep relaxation just after eating a heavy meal. Many people also find that deep relaxation just before sleep can lead to a restless night. This is because, after deep relaxation, your body becomes naturally more awake and alert for a time. Taking about 15 minutes to occur, this alertness will then last for several hours. When you finish a relaxation session, bring yourself around slowly — it's best to avoid setting an alarm, as the shock can undo all the benefits you've achieved.

Focused breathing and progressive muscle relaxation are two commonly used and effective deep relaxation techniques.

Focused breathing

This is an extremely easy technique needing very little effort that allows your body's natural rhythms to take over. It's not a fierce, forced concentration, but a relaxed, easy attention. And the moments when you drift away from it are an important part of the process. The only real "discipline" required is in bringing your attention back when you notice it has wandered.

One of the benefits of focused breathing is that it can be done in almost any setting, in any clothes, without making a song and dance out of it. And with practice, you'll find that even a few minutes can be refreshing. Although not strictly necessary, if you're physically tense it may help to set the stage with some light stretching before you sit. You can even combine this method with the technique of progressive relaxation. Do the progressive relaxation first, then move into focused breathing.

To practice focused breathing, sit in a comfortable chair with your eyes closed. The exact sitting position doesn't matter, as long as you can remain comfortable for 10 or 20 minutes. Consciously relax any obviously tense muscles. Then turn your attention to your breath.

The key to this method is to observe your breathing without changing it at all. You don't need to breathe in any particular way — let your body breathe, and simply observe the breath. As you continue to do this, a moment will come when you realize that you're no longer observing your breath — simply return your attention to your breath. Do this as often as necessary, for as long as you think useful.

Progressive muscle relaxation

This technique is based on a simple physiological principle: if you tense a muscle, the muscle will relax more deeply when you release the contraction. By contracting and releasing your muscles one after the other, you can bring your entire body to a state of deep relaxation in about five minutes. Adrenaline junkies in particular might find progressive muscular relaxation useful.

The relaxation is most easily done lying down but you can also do it sitting. Start with your right foot. Tense the foot, contracting the toes, the sole and the top of the foot. Hold the contraction and take a deep breath in. Release the breath and release the muscle contraction simultaneously.

Now tense your calf and shin, and release. Then move to the thigh (front and back), the hips and buttock. Repeat for your left leg. Continue through the rest of your body in the following order: right hand, right forearm, right upper arm and the same for your left arm; then lower back, abdomen, upper back, chest, shoulders, neck and face.

Do this process slowly. Hold each contraction for a couple of seconds while you inhale slowly, then release the tension and breathe for about a second. Take a couple of breaths before moving to the next part of your body.

When you've finished contracting and releasing all your muscles, continue to lie still for another five or ten minutes. Do nothing but relax.

high stress

Your chemistry is there to help your body under stress. Adrenaline fires to push you through with a cortisol backup if the stress continues for most of the day. Serotonin is a buffer to depression and ensures calm. If stress is prolonged or unusually high your chemistry will show it, so when you improve how you deal with stress you'll have balanced body chemistry.

1 The best performance is achieved by being neither totally relaxed nor totally aroused.

2 Stress thresholds are measures of how much stress you can tolerate before your performance or health is affected.

3 Anything that has an impact on you, for good or bad, causes stress. If the accumulated stress passes your threshold, it affects you adversely.

4 Your body has a mechanism for relaxation just as it has a mechanism for arousal (the flight or fight response). Like a car, you can "change gears" between a high power mode and a cruising or idling mode. Taking charge of this process will enhance your health and improve your performance.

5 Tasks that require more precision or thinking are best done when the body is more relaxed. Tasks that are more physical, and less precise, work well with more arousal. High arousal gives sparkle or vigor to your performance but can also cause verbal or physical clumsiness.

6 The relaxation response restores balance and replenishes energy stores. It supports essential maintenance activities such as digestion and repair.

7 Deep relaxation is not useful in dealing with a crisis but helps prepare for a crisis, and for dealing with the after-effects of the crisis on your system.

> We must not, in trying to think about how we can make a big difference, ignore the small daily differences we can make which, over time, add up to big differences that we often cannot foresee.
>
> MARIAN WRIGHT EDELMAN

11

the high life plan

the high life plan

Achieving a naturally high life involves three steps:

<1> doing a lifestyle audit

<2> filling in the current personal chemical profile

<3> learning to navigate your highways

step 1 > the lifestyle audit

The five lifestyle keys of sleep, food, exercise, thoughts and stress are listed below. Take a few moments to review the quality of each in your life right now. Then write down one action you think would help you improve this lifestyle key. Take note of which lifestyle area needs an overhaul and make any common sense moves toward fixing that imbalance.

SLEEP

How are you sleeping at the moment?

❍ poorly ❍ average ❍ well

What can you do immediately that would make a difference to how well you sleep?

____

____

____

You may decide to:

1. Go to bed at the same time each night
2. Sleep in natural fibers
3. Buy a new pillow
4. Install air-conditioning or fans to even out temperature
5. Install an air filter by your bed
6. Read in bed with a mini light to reduce stimulation
7. Remove the television from the bedroom
8. Rotate the mattress
9. Shake your duvet to even out the down
10. Buy a king size bed
11. Drink a cup of camomile tea before bed
12. Use candles in the bathroom as you prepare for bed
13. Put dimmer switches on all the lights and dim the lights a little every 30 minutes from sundown
14. Exercise in the middle of the day
15. Get outside away from fluorescent lighting during the day

FOOD

What is your diet like at the moment?

❍ terrible ❍ alright ❍ fantastic

What can you do immediately to improve your nutrition?

___

___

___

You may decide to:

1. Drink at least eight cups of water a day
2. Snack on dried fruit or trail mix
3. Eat more turkey and almonds
4. Pre-prepare salad boxes as quick lunches or dinner side dishes
5. Eat fish three times a week
6. Buy a blender and make your own juices and smoothies
7. Have a low-fat, high-protein breakfast two to three times a week
8. Drink decaffeinated skim milk coffees
9. Drink less than three alcoholic drinks a day and have alcohol-free days each week
10. Take a multivitamin each day
11. Eat more low GI foods
12. Eat lots of fiber-rich foods and control hunger
13. Eat every four waking hours
14. Always eat breakfast
15. Buy organic foods and avoid highly processed meals

ACTIVITY

Are you active and exercising?

❍ no ❍ mostly ❍ yes

What can you do immediately to be more active or get more exercise into your day?

___

___

___

You may decide to:

1. Ask a friend to walk with you at lunchtime
2. Pack a bag of clothes and exercise gear each night so it's automatically ready the next day
3. Exercise in the morning before breakfast to burn fat
4. Exercise at lunchtime to improve sleep at night
5. Exercise in the early evening to reduce stress
6. Build lean muscle to control sugar highs and lows by doing weights
7. Get rid of cortisol and anxiety by doing vigorous or tough exercise
8. Swim laps or join a swim club
9. Choose a local exercise event, such as a fun run, and challenge yourself to get fit in time for the event
10. Check out a gym and join if it's right for you
11. Rediscover a childhood sport
12. Buy a heavy-duty, off-road stroller, or baby back carrier, and do some serious walking with baby
13. Take up yoga
14. Start or join a walking group
15. Do some stretching and calisthenics each day as you wake before getting ready for your day

THOUGHTS

How would you rate your thought processes?

❍ negative ❍ bit of both ❍ positive

What can you do immediately to improve your thought habits?

____

____

____

You may decide to:

1. Keep a journal so you can witness your thoughts and get to know what's going on in your head
2. Buy some positive thinking tapes and listen to them in the car to and from work
3. Make a list of loose ends or unresolved issues and methodically seek closure on them
4. Make friends with people supportive of your desired life and change those who are not
5. Enroll in creativity workshops, seeking diversity to expand your ideas
6. Avoid speed talking and thinking and affirm abundance rather than lack
7. Focus your mind on today and what's happening around you, rather than thinking anxiously about the past or future
8. Aim to build your self-esteem through education — read self-development books or attend workshops and seminars
9. Make the reason for doing things more personal and driven less from approval or feedback
10. Make comedy a steady part of your life by subscribing to the comedy channel, renting videos or DVDs of comedians or going to see live stand-up comedians
11. Always seek flexibility of thought and watch out for rigid thinking patterns
12. Beware of cynicism and remember that not every experience has a negative
13. Be clear on what you want in life so you can say "no" to those things you don't want
14. Stop being a perfectionist — a desire for perfection is often an attempt to control your outside world to make up for a lack on the inside
15. Capture the learning from every challenge and document this somehow

STRESS

How high is your stress level at the moment?

❍ low ❍ moderate ❍ high

What can you do immediately that would make a difference to your level of stress?

____

____

____

You may decide to:

1. Eliminate some activities and simplify your life
2. Schedule in days off and plan vacations at least 90 days ahead
3. Do some vigorous exercise at the end of the day to burn off the stress chemical cortisol
4. Enroll in a meditation course
5. Invest in a regular (weekly) massage session
6. Enroll in a meditation course
7. Make an absolute priority list of ten things that you will always say "yes" to
8. Do the most important things at the start of your day, then if the day flies by you will have achieved something
9. Make a coffee shop appointment, or time-out appointment, with yourself each day. Use this 10 minutes to half an hour to read the paper, plan your day or simply relax
10. Attend a time management or personal effectiveness course
11. Become assertive and eliminate waste-of-time meetings or phone calls
12. Do something spontaneous
13. Break the routine. Drive a different way to work or eat somewhere different
14. Decide that when work is finished for the day it's finished — don't go back to it later
15. Stay focused on what people are saying rather than disconnecting and thinking about something else

step 2 > your current personal chemical profile

Each time you do your current personal chemical profile you'll get a different picture of the chemicals on which you're running. When everything is going well your profile will be balanced. When things are out of balance, or you're under a lot of stress, it will show on your profile.

Adrenaline

1 Do you find yourself eating more quickly than others around you? ❍ yes ❍ no
2 Would you eat lunch at your desk more than 3 times a week? ❍ yes ❍ no
3 Do you often drive fast even if you're not in a hurry? ❍ yes ❍ no
4 If you had 3 weeks to finish something would you still leave it until the last minute? ❍ yes ❍ no
5 Is it hard to imagine yourself doing nothing? Just sitting — no TV, no reading, absolutely nothing — for an hour a day? ❍ yes ❍ no

YOUR SCORE ❑ yes ❑ no

If you answered "yes" to more than 3 of these questions you're probably an adrenaline junkie.

Serotonin

1 Do you find that a cloudy day affects your disposition? ❍ yes ❍ no
2 Do you eat after you've had an argument? ❍ yes ❍ no
3 Do you crave sugar mid-afternoon? ❍ yes ❍ no
4 Do you snack mainly on carbohydrates rather than proteins? ❍ yes ❍ no
5 When stressed, are you likely to have mood swings? ❍ yes ❍ no

YOUR SCORE ❑ yes ❑ no

If you answered "yes" to more than 3 of these questions you're probably a serotonin seeker.

Cortisol

1 Can you imagine driving home, thinking loving thoughts about your kids, only to yell at one of them when you walk through the door? ❍ yes ❍ no
2 Do you think you snap at people more than you should? ❍ yes ❍ no
3 If you're a regular exerciser and miss a workout for a couple of days, do you feel a creeping edginess? ❍ yes ❍ no
4 Do you often find yourself twitching and foot tapping in meetings where you're required to listen rather than speak? ❍ yes ❍ no

5 When stressed, do you become angry, sad, afraid or guilty more often than you think you should? ❍ yes ❍ no

YOUR SCORE ❑ yes ❑ no

If you answered "yes" to more than 3 of these questions you're probably getting cranky on cortisol.

Melatonin

1 If you drink coffee in the evening do you feel it affects the quality of your sleep? ❍ yes ❍ no
2 When you spend a day in the sun do you sleep better at night? ❍ yes ❍ no
3 If you're stressed during your day, do you find it hard to sleep well at night? ❍ yes ❍ no
4 Do you think you suffer from jet lag more than other people you travel with? ❍ yes ❍ no
5 Would you love to travel with your own bed and pillow whenever you were away from home? ❍ yes ❍ no

YOUR SCORE ❑ yes ❑ no

If you answered "yes" to more than 3 of these questions you probably need to increase melatonin levels.

Insulin and sugar sensitivity

1 Do you find you're sleepy after lunch more often than not? ❍ yes ❍ no
2 Does a sweet snack give you a noticeable rush or temporary high? ❍ yes ❍ no
3 Is your day a roller coaster of energy and mood — one moment you can focus with great clarity and the next moment you're clueless? ❍ yes ❍ no
4 Are you tired a lot of the time? ❍ yes ❍ no
5 Does your attention wander? Do you have trouble concentrating, particularly when stressed? ❍ yes ❍ no

YOUR SCORE ❑ yes ❑ no

If you answered "yes" to more than 3 of these questions you may have a sugar sensitivity.

step 3 > navigating your highways

Your current personal chemical profile should highlight which of the 5 key chemicals you're either running on or are deficient in. Look for those chemicals that have three or more yes answers. Your profile could look more like Phillip's or Katerina's.

Phillip's current personal chemical profile

Adrenaline	5 yes	0 no
Serotonin	2 yes	3 no
Cortisol	3 yes	2 no
Melatonin	0 yes	5 no
Insulin	0 yes	5 no

Katerina's current personal chemical profile

Adrenaline	1 yes	4 no
Serotonin	1 yes	4 no
Cortisol	1 yes	4 no
Melatonin	5 yes	0 no
Insulin	1 yes	4 no

Phillip is high adrenaline (5 yes answers) with a secondary cortisol profile (3 yes answers). He needs to look at the adrenaline and cortisol navigation points and go to work on those areas only. Katerina, on the other hand, only needs to focus on sleep and balancing her melatonin system. The customized prescription makes strategies for greater motivation and less stress more relevant and effective. The result? A naturally high life!

NAVIGATING THE ADRENALINE EXPRESSWAY

‹1› Learn to read the adrenaline road signs

When you're on adrenaline your body will give you clues through changes in breathing and heart rate, and a drop in body temperature, particularly the feet and hands.

Avoid shallow, sharp breaths, slow down under stress and breathe more deeply. Learn how to take your heart rate and monitor it throughout the day. If you find it's 20 beats per minute above your resting heart rate, and you're not exercising, adrenaline is probably present. Learn to read the signs of adrenaline and then either use it and push through, or consciously slow down and spare the adrenaline.

‹2› Prioritize adrenaline events

If you're always running late or working with urgency and constantly putting pressure on yourself, you run the risk of depleting adrenaline stores and becoming out of balance.

Look at the events in your day and decide if it's an Adrenaline Priority Event (APE). Sometimes it's appropriate to go APE and sometimes an event just doesn't warrant the use of this precious fuel. If you have a crisis and need to use adrenaline, go for it! Deadlines, emergencies at work, looking after a sick child and important projects require a certain push. Adrenaline, and what it provides, help you through these times. Giving a presentation is an adrenaline priority event, being late for a meeting is not. Imagine that you have three hours of adrenaline a day at your disposal and use that store on Adrenaline Priority Events.

3 Build a strong heart

Adrenaline places a demand on your circulatory system, causing your blood to thicken.

If adrenaline plays a significant part in your current chemical profile, make aerobic exercise a priority to keep your heart strong.

4 Send the message "all's well"

When you eat you send a message that all is well. But when you skip meals your body thinks you're in trouble and releases adrenaline.

Eat breakfast and then continue to eat every four hours. Eating is the quickest way to reassure your body that the stress can't be all that bad. When you don't eat, everything becomes a stress event.

5 Slow down everyday activities

If you do everything in fast forward a stressed life will evolve into a burned out one.

You need to step off speed and make some space in your life. When you leave work, drive in silence or come prepared to read on the bus or listen to a CD. Then read for an hour or so when you get home before you switch on the TV. If you find yourself nodding off, go to bed a little earlier — you'll sleep through the night more often. You may still want to watch an hour or so of TV after reading, but the initial pause from TV's stimulation is just enough for your body to tell you of its need for sleep. If you're coming home to a rush hour with kids, try to take a moment for yourself earlier in the day.

6 Switch off and brain dump

Switching off at night is difficult for adrenaline junkies — you stimulate yourself by thinking in loops. Then often just as you're about to drop off you start to think of the most creative and innovative things.

Slow down during the day so you have access to this creative process at a more convenient time. At night, try brain dumping, for example, speaking into a dictaphone to get the idea out of your head, or keeping a note pad by your bed and jotting down the ideas. Whatever you choose as your method, you need to get the thoughts out of your head and onto something tangible so you can review the idea when you wake. If you don't you'll loop unproductively around and around the same idea.

NAVIGATING THE SEROTONIN ROUNDABOUT

‹1› Control cravings

Your craving or hunger for something sweet, particularly in the early afternoons, is a crude message from your brain to get more serotonin.

Pause before responding and choose your food. The solution is a small dose of sugar (40 grams). To minimize the hunger responses, eat more fiber and reduce highly processed foods. Protein is also a craving neutral food and eating some protein with most meals will slow down many cravings.

‹2› Do easy exercise

The human body was made to move and the dramatic decrease in physical activity in the past few decades is causing severe chemical imbalances.

Evidence suggests that easy exercise elevates serotonin and decreases depression. Working out every other day, going for a walk, swimming some laps, playing with the dog or hitting a round of golf will help balance your body chemistry.

‹3› Take a break

As you burn out and hit the natural "lows" of low serotonin, you begin to lose interest in what you're doing.

Take a break and program some pause into your day, then identify how often you need that pause. Have a hobby for mini breaks and don't eat lunch at your desk. Consider enrolling in a course, having a holiday at home, planning a long weekend or not answering the phone for a weekend. By investing in a little rest you'll reap a huge return in increased focus, passion and productivity.

‹4› Monitor your thinking

When your thinking has become distorted, or you've become inflexible, judgmental, irrational and blowing things out of all proportion, you're suffering from stinking thinking.

You need to take responsibility for making changes in your life and learn how to grow out of the thought traps you set for yourself.

‹5› Eat more meat

The blood around the brain needs to be cleared with controlled sugar hits — but most people overdose on sugar in response to a craving and end up asleep or lacking energy as insulin rages through the system in response to the huge sugar dump.

Turkey, red meat and almonds are just a few of the foods rich in tryptophan, the basic protein from which your brain manufactures serotonin. Eating these every other day ensures you have enough protein available for the brain to manufacture happy chemicals. If you eat foods rich in tryptophan, each day also have a controlled sugar hit and wait 20 minutes for the serotonin to kick in. Ideal hits include 1/3 cup of raisins or two bananas.

6 Get touched regularly

Therapeutic massage has been shown to have a positive effect on those with mild depression. The regular physical contact increases calm, and decreases anger and anxiety by stimulating the serotonin system.

If you're not being touched regularly, consider paying for a professional massage. Pets can also be good touch therapy.

NAVIGATING CORTISOL GRIDLOCK

1 Manage your accumulated stress

When everything in life becomes a stress event, it's a sign that cortisol has taken over. If you find yourself "losing it" it's often because the pressure of the day builds up, even if it started calmly.

Think back and try to identify any unnecessary overreactions earlier in the day — you may have been going so fast you forgot to ask yourself whether the issue was really worth the angst. So stop before every reaction and ask what would be the best thing to do or say right now. Pause!

2 Laugh a lot

Under stress it's easy to lose your sense of humor, yet humor is the ideal weapon for combating stress — it's not possible to laugh and have high cortisol. So subscribe to the comedy channel, rent funny videos and go to live stand-up comedy shows.

3 Take care with stimulants

Stimulants such as licorice (which prevents the breakdown of cortisol), caffeine and nicotine keep you on edge.

Although useful if you're trying to stay "on" during an important event, or to help you work through the night, stimulants will prevent you from relaxing. So if your profile has high cortisol, you need to limit or eliminate these substances.

4 Do vigorous exercise

Vigorous or tough exercise helps counter the increased muscular tension of stress and reduces cortisol levels, resulting in a calm feeling.

If you've had a particularly tough day, go for a jog, stop at the gym or walk briskly around the block to cool down before you greet your loved ones.

5 Develop extreme respect

When you're cortisol crazy you become snappy and short tempered with others.

While it won't reduce your cortisol response, a polite respectful orientation toward others will hide the crazy feeling. This gives you time to control the rage and choose to fly off the handle or not — you'll regret the Jekyll-and-Hyde act within the hour. So keep in the front of your mind that everyone is doing the best they can with what they have.

NAVIGATING THE MELATONIN OFF RAMP

1 Get plenty of natural light by day and use darkness at night

Artificial lighting, while generally not bright enough to turn on serotonin, is bright enough to prevent melatonin production. When it gets dark your brain begins to release melatonin so you sleep deeply. If you stay indoors during the day and keep bright lights and wide screen TVs blasting through your retinas at night, melatonin is prevented from doing its job.

Get outside as often as you can. This signals the pineal gland to manufacture melatonin, which will help you sleep better at night. If you want deeper sleep you also need to shut out light at night — the darker you can make the bedroom the better, as daylight sends a trigger to your brain to switch off melatonin production and begin manufacturing serotonin. Put dimmer switches on every light in the house and after dark turn the lights down. Use candles in the bathroom at night and read using a mini book light, or at least use low watt light bulbs in your reading lamps.

2 Establish a routine

The more regular you are with your sleep and wake times the more in tune your body clock is to your needs — you'll be awake in the day when you need to be and tired at night when you need to be.

Get to love routine, especially if you have a strong tendency toward melatonin in your personal chemical profile. Go to bed at set times and wake up at set times. Exercise at the same time every day. Eat regular meals and eat them at the same time each day. Give your body clock every possible chance to match your routines so you can be on during the day when you should be and off at night as you would expect.

3 Exercise in the day, relax at night

Research has shown that you'll sleep better at night if you exercise during the day, particularly aerobic exercise.

So if you don't sleep well at night, think seriously about taking a brisk walk or light jog as part of your lunchtime plan. Exercise during the day will help your body know its sleep–wake cycle and should help reduce nighttime restlessness caused by a still active serotonin system.

‹4› Relax before going to bed

Before electricity there was a natural downturn before going to sleep as you were limited in what you could do when it was dark.

Rediscover that drop off in activity, learn to wind down before going to bed. Read a book, listen to soothing music or have a warm bath before you go to bed and only use your bed for sleeping. Avoid stimulants including tobacco, alcohol, tea, coffee or chocolate for at least four hours before sleep. Minimize your caffeine to less than 300 mg a day or about five cups of filtered coffee — this can bring about a huge shift in the balance of your body chemistry. If it's just the taste of coffee you love, have a decaffeinated coffee (the caffeine content is less than 1 mg per cup).

‹5› Regulate your body temperature in bed

Your depth of sleep will be affected by your own body temperature as well as that of your partner.

To help maintain a consistent body temperature when you sleep, shake out your bed covering before you lie down so that the down and feathers are evenly distributed. Also have different summer and winter bed covers if your seasonal temperatures vary greatly and wear nightwear made from natural fibers that breathe, such as cotton.

If you sleep with your partner, cuddle them then dispatch them to their side of the bed. If you're both heavier than 130 pounds, consider a king size bed so you can each retreat to your corners and get a good night's sleep. Consider separate bed covers if you and your partner are typically different temperatures when in bed.

NAVIGATING THE INSULIN CRASH ZONE

‹1› Avoid refined and quickly digested sugars

Cutting back on refined and quickly digested sugars will moderate insulin responses and balance blood sugar levels.

Avoid those sugars that quickly enter your blood, such as too much white rice, white bread or highly processed sugar based foods. Slowly digested sugars are those that are rough and chewy, and closest to their natural form as possible. Good choices include pasta over rice, apples over bananas, or dried apricots and strawberries whenever you want.

‹2› Exercise to moderate blood sugar levels

For about 30 minutes after exercise, any sugars you eat, whether they be quickly or slowly digested, are stored as fuel and insulin release is suppressed.

If you exercise in the mornings and feel tired throughout the rest of the day, eating during the 30 minutes post exercise may help your energy levels.

Weight training will also help balance sugar levels and excessive insulin responses. The more lean muscle tissue you have the more excess sugar you can store, and the less sensitive you'll be to sugar and the subsequent insulin reactions.

3 Eat more protein

Of the three major nutrients (fats, carbohydrates and proteins), protein is the only one that doesn't create an insulin response.

Shifting to a protein-rich diet can help you focus, increase energy levels and control weight. Eat lean proteins like fish, grilled chicken and lean cuts of meat or search for vegetarian proteins like low-fat tofu, beans and legumes.

4 Lose weight

If you're overweight you force your insulin system to work overtime. Lose weight and you'll reduce the insulin crashes.

5 Eat small meals often

Insulin responds to large amounts of sugar. Eating smaller meals more often (grazing) prevents this. While you're awake try to eat every four hours rather than going for hours before you think of food.

the high life

High life is about increasing your choices so you can feel uplifted 24 hours a day 7 days a week. To do this, you need to be vigilant for burnout indicators or signs of lifestyle imbalance through your current chemical profile. Every 90 days, redo your profile and notice any new imbalances, then make the specific changes suggested in this book for each of the 5 key chemicals.

By making adjustments to the tangible areas of sleep, food and physical activity, you'll begin to see immediate changes in the quality of your life. You'll feel more energetic, less stressed, more capable and you'll be in a generally higher state than before. Focusing on how you think and managing stress more effectively will result in fewer of life's low points.

No matter how high or how low your life is right now, you can make small changes and maximize your body's key chemicals. You, too, can achieve a natural high.

So take good care of your own lawn and lead a naturally high life!

When the grass looks greener on the

other side of the fence, it may be that

they are taking better care of it.

CECIL SELIG

references

3 adrenaline junkies

Church, M. 1999, *Adrenaline Junkies – The Chemistry of Success*, Live Life Publications

Gold, P.W. 1998, "Clinical and Biological Manifestations of Depression," *New England Journal of Medicine*, 319:413-419

Hart, A. 1995, *Adrenaline and Stress*, Word Publishing

Jennings, J. & Haughton, L. 2000, *It's Not the Big That Eat the Small, It's the Fast That Eat the Slow – How to Use Speed as a Competitive Tool,* Harper Business

4 serotonin seekers

Aldridge, S. 2000, *Seeing Red and Feeling Blue: The New Understanding of Mood and Emotion*, Arrow Books Random House

Barker, R. 1997, *Baby Love: Everything You Need to Know about Your New Baby*, Pan Macmillan

Comings, D.E. 1994, "Serotonin: A Key to Migraine Disorders," *Nutrition Health Review* 70:6

DesMaisons, K. 1996, *Potatoes Not Prozac*, Simon & Schuster

Linnoila, M. 1983, "Low cerebrospinal fluid 5-hydroxy-indoleacetic acid concentration differentiates impulsive from non impulsive violent behaviour," *Life Science*, 33:2609-2614

5 unnatural high

Bell, I.R. 1991, "B Complex Vitamin Patterns in Geriatric and Young Adult Inpatients with Major Depression," *Journal of American Geriatric Society*, 39:252-257

Jacobs, B.L. 1991, "Serotonin and Behaviour: Emphasis on Motor Control," *Journal of Clinical Psychiatry* 51, suppl. 12

Kasper, S. 1997, "Treatment of Seasonal Affective Disorder (SAD) with Hypericum Extract," *Pharmacopsychiatry*, vol. 30:89-93

Seelig, M. 1992, "Adverse Stress Reactions and Magnesium Deficiency: Preventative and Therapeutic Implications," *Journal of American College of Nutrition*, 11(5):609

Swan, G. & Carmelli, D. 1995, "Characteristics Associated with Excessive Weight Gain after Smoking Cessation in Men," *American Journal of Public Health*, 85(1):73-77

Volz, H.P. 1997, "Controlled Clinical Trials of Hypericum Extracts in Out-patients an Overview," *Pharmacopsychiatry*, vol. 3, suppl. 2

6 deep sleep

Coren, S. 1996, *Sleep Thieves*, The Free Press

Mass, J.B. 1998, *Power Sleep: The Revolutionary Program That Prepares Your Mind for Peak Performance*, Villard

Sagan, C. 1996, *The Demon Haunted World: Science as a Candle in the Dark*, Ballantine Books

7 mood foods

Egger, G. 1995, "Is Alcohol Fattening? Findings from the 7th International Congress on Obesity," *Gut Busters: Waist Watch*, No. 10

Fernstrom, J.D. & Wurtman, R.J. 1971, "Brain Serotonin: Increase Following Ingestion of Carbohydrate Diet," *Science* 174:1023-1025

Macdiarmid, J. & Hetherington, M. 1995, "Mood Modulation by Food: An Exploration of Affect and Cravings in 'Chocolate Addicts,'" *British Journal of Clinical Psychology*, 34 (Pt.1):129-138

National Health and Nutrition Examination Survey (NHANES) 1992, "Depression Effects on Weight Gain," *International Journal of Obesity*,16:745-753

Rosmond, R. 2000, "Food Induced Cortisol Secretion in Relation to Metabolic and Haemodynamic Variables in Men," *International Journal of Obesity*, 24:416-422

Stanton, R. 1994, *Eating For Peak Performance*, Allen & Unwin

Weltzin, T. E., Fernstrom, J.D. & Kaye W.H. 1995, "Serotonin and Bulimia Nervosa," *American Journal of Psychiatry*,152:1668-1672

Young, S.N. 1996, "Behavioural Effects of Dietary Neurotransmitter Precursors: Basic and Clinical Aspects," *Neuroscience and Biobehavioural Reviews*, vol. 20, no. 2:313-323

8 Churchill's urge

Egger, G. & Champion, N. 1999, *The Fitness Leaders Handbook*, Kangaroo Press

Fox, E. & Mathews, D. 1976, *The Physiological Basis of Physical Education and Athletics, W.B. Saunders & Co.*

Helms, D. & Turner, S. 1987, *Lifespan Development*, Harcourt Brace Jovanovich International

9 mind over matter

Adrienne, C. 1998, *The Purpose of Your Life*, Eagle Brook

Atkinson, R.L., Atkinson, R.C. & Hilgard, E. 1981, *Introduction to Psychology*, Harcourt Brace Jovanovich International

Roger, J. & McWilliams, P. 1991, *Do It! A Guide to Living Your Dreams*, Thorsons

Sagan, C. & Druyan, A. 1992, *Shadows of Forgotten Ancestors: A Search for Who We Are*, Random House

Selegam, M.E.P. 1990, *Learned Optimism: Optimism Is Essential for a Good and Successful Life. You Too Can Acquire It*, Random House

Solso, R.L. 1997, *Mind and Brain Sciences in the 21st Century*, Bradford Press MIT

10 high stress

Holmes, T. & Rahe, R.H. 1967, "The Social Readjustment Rating Scale," *Journal of Psychosomatic Research* II:213-218

Maslac, C. & Leiter, M. 1997, *The Truth about Burnout: How Organizations Cause Personal Stress and What to Do About It,* Jossey-Bass Publishers

Seyle, H. 1956, *The Stress Of Life*, McGraw Hill

Hanson, P. 1989, *Stress For Success*, Collins

Thanks to the whole team at ABC books for their commitment to making *Highlife* a great book. I would especially like to thank my commissioning editor Jill Brown for having the ability to sit in a room and visualize this book while I was speaking. Thanks also to my editor Patricia Hoyle for her patient and well-considered work. The book is so much better because of you. Finally, I'm grateful to Melanie Feddersen for her inspired and elegant design.

Thanks also to Wendy Church and Patricia Hughes who edited the first draft. That's what mums and best friends do, isn't it? And my biggest thanks to my wife Lex, who put up with my mental and physical absence from the things we normally do while this book came together.

thank you

Matt Church has a BSc in Applied Science from the University of New South Wales in Australia. He started his career in the fitness industry, and then was a lecturer and program developer for the Australian Council of Health and Physical Education and Recreation. He is now one of Australia's leading conference speakers. His uplifting seminar series, *The Chemistry of Success*, leaves people from a diverse range of industries feeling recharged and motivated to improve their personal chemical profile. *Adrenaline Junkies & Serotonin Seekers* is a distillation of years of researching and presenting on the topics of work/life balance, body chemistry and managing stress.

about matt

other ulysses press books

Belly Dancing for Fitness: The Ultimate Dance Workout That Unleashes Your Creative Spirit
Tamalyn Dallal with Richard Harris, $14.95
Drawing from her years of experience as a world-famous teacher and performer, the author carefully leads the reader through each skill level of this increasingly popular exercises art form.

Ellie Herman's Pilates Props Workbook: Step-by-Step Guide with over 350 Photos
Ellie Herman, $14.95
Introduces the reader to popular workout accessories that amplify Pilates matwork exercises.

Workouts from Boxing's Greatest Champs
Gary Todd, $14.95
This unique approach allows you to devise a training program based on the regimens of the champs but tailored to suit your fitness goals.

Yoga in Focus: Postures, Sequences, and Meditations
Jessie Chapman photographs by Dhyan, $14.95
A beautiful celebration of yoga that's both useful for learning the techniques and inspiring in its artistic approach to presenting the body in yoga positions.

To order these books call 800-377-2542 or 510-601-8301, fax 510-601-8307, e-mail ulysses@ulyssespress.com, or write to Ulysses Press, P.O. Box 3440, Berkeley, CA 94703. All retail orders are shipped free of charge. California residents must include sales tax. Allow two to three weeks for delivery.

other books